CORONA DEMYSTIFIED

CORONA FORMULAS
CORONA TABLES
CORONA BRAKE

Know it to beat it

Jacob Sebastian

MS, MIE, MBA.

INTERNATIONAL EDITION

CORONA DEMYSTIFIED
CORONA FORMULAS, CORONA TABLES, OMICRON BRAKE.
January 2022

Author: **Jacob Sebastian**

jacobsebastian@highwaytoriches.info

www.highwaytoriches.info

Copyright © 2022 by **Jacob Sebastian**

DISCLAIMER

ISBN: 978 908 3120 379

Dekkaan Publishing, Rotterdam, The Netherlands, EU.

ABOUT THE AUTHOR

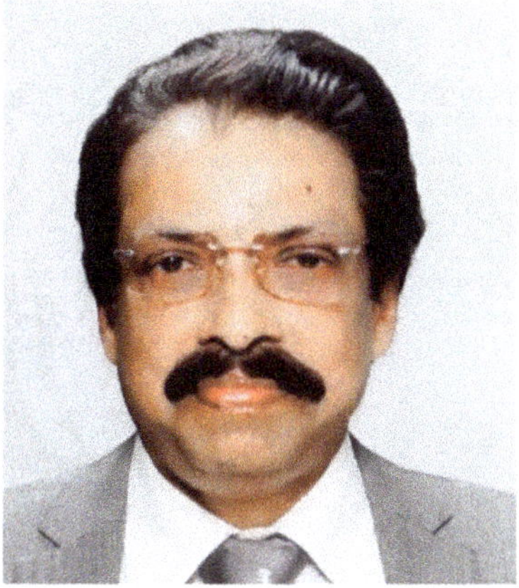

Jacob Sebastian is an engineer, born in India and a citizen of the Netherlands (EU). His academic credentials include the following:

- Graduation in Mechanical Engineering (India).
- Postgraduation in Combustion Technology (IIT Madras, India).
- Postgraduation in Energy Management (Netherlands).
- MBA in International Trade and Finance (UK).

He has held senior engineering and management positions with the Government of India, an industrial conglomerate in the Middle East, and the European Division of a US-based Fortune-500 corporation. Subsequently, he established and operated his own software development and real estate development businesses.

He has received several achievement awards, excelling in academic, professional, and business fields. As chief engineer of a major industrial concern in the Netherlands, he has achieved a reduction of 300 million kg of global-warming CO2 emission through innovation.

He has published a book in 2021 titled "Compounding, the Wizard of Wealth Building," which is an in-depth guide to all aspects of compound interest and exponential growth of wealth.

He lives in Rotterdam, The Netherlands (EU). He can be reached at:

jacobsebastian@highwaytoriches.info

www.highwaytoriches.info

TABLE OF CONTENTS

1   INTRODUCTION

Starting in December 2019 in Wuhan, China, with one person infected, the virus had spread to all countries in the world and infected about **285 million** people and caused about **5.4 million deaths** by the end of 2021, two years from the start of the pandemic.

Mathematically, the Covid-19 pandemic is probably the most widespread and maliciously impactful process of compounding and exponential growth that humanity has faced in the last hundred years. Therefore, the pandemic has made the subject of compounding more relevant than it has ever been before.

During the past two years, when I was busy preparing my book titled "Compounding, the Wizard of Wealth Building," which was initially intended to enable readers to utilize the power of compounding to build wealth bigger and faster, the pandemic emerged and subsequently took the whole world in its stranglehold. Unfortunately, against all hopes that the pandemic would be a short-lived disaster that would disappear quickly, it has become clear that it is here for a more extended stay.

From a mathematical point of view, the growth of Covid-19 infections in the community is nothing other than compounding and the resultant exponential growth. Therefore, I have added a special chapter titled "Covid-19 Pandemic and Compounding" to the second edition of my book "Compounding, the Wizard of Wealth Building" that has just been published. This book is an extended version of that chapter, elaborated and supplemented with additional information and tables.

This book contains a rather detailed analysis of the virus's infection, replication, and transmission from a mathematical point of view, hopefully filling a knowledge gap that will help us beat the virus. The focus is specifically on the growth and spread of the **Delta** and **Omicron** variants. In addition, the replication and growth of virus particles in the human body are also looked at from a mathematical perspective to increase our understanding of what happens when we get infected.

The two main factors that determine the spread of Covid-19 are the **Reproduction rate R** and the **Generation speed G**. The factor by which Covid-19 infections increase weekly in a community is given by the formula R^G.

The impact of this unholy bond between R & G is analyzed in detail, and a singular way to make this devious couple virtually impotent and incapable of spreading fast through exponential growth is discussed. This fundamentally mathematical knowledge is essential to curbing the spread of the virus, especially the speedy variants like Omicron or any speedier future variants.

The **Corona Table** is the summmum of this book. It contains the mathematically expected growth rates of Covid-19 infections with Omicron, Delta, and the original version of the virus for a range of Reproduction numbers, from 0.70 to 10.0. If one person gets infected, the table shows the actual number of new infections per week, the week-to-week growth factor, month-to-month growth factor, the daily growth rate in %, the doubling time of new infections in days and hours, and the days and hours needed to reduce new infections to half the prevailing rate when the pandemic is on retreat.

* * * *

2   SOME BASIC DEFINITIONS & DATA

Incubation period: It is the period between the moment of getting infected and the moment of getting symptoms or feeling sick. The average incubation period is about **7 days** for the original version, **5 days** for Delta, and **3.5 days** for Omicron.

The incubation period takes very long for some people and ends without developing any symptoms. But in the meantime, they have also been infectious for some time, like others who do develop symptoms. That makes them "blind" spreaders.

Latent period: It is the period between getting infected and becoming infectious and potentially infecting others. The average latent period is reported to be about **4 days** for the original version, **2 days** for Delta, and **1 day** for Omicron.

For Covid-19, the latent period ends, and the infectious period starts about **2 days** before the Incubation period ends and symptoms appear. This overlap of 2 days makes these infected persons "blind" spreaders without being aware that they are infected.

It is reported that 44% of all Omicron infections occur in the undetected 2-day gap between the start of the infectious period and the start of symptoms. Infecting others in this period is entirely logical from a mathematical perspective, as explained later in this book.

Transmission period or Infectious period: It is the period in which an infected person can shed the virus and potentially infect others. By definition, it starts at the end of the Latent Period and lasts until all the symptoms of illness have disappeared. It is from **day-3 to day-10 for Delta** and **day-2 to day-10 for Omicron.**

Period of Maximum Transmissibility or Infectiousness: For Delta, it is reported to be from **day-3 to day-7,** with the **peak** lying at around **5 days**. For Omicron, it is estimated to be from **day-2 to day-7,** with the **peak** lying at around **4 days.** For severely ill patients, the period can be much longer.

Generation Time or Generation Period: It is the average time between one person getting infected and he, in turn, infecting another person. It was about **7 days** for the original version in early 2020. It is only about **5 days for Delta** and is estimated to be only **3.5 days for Omicron**.

Generation Speed G: It is the inverse of Generation Time and is measured as the number of **Generations per week**. It was **1.0** Generation per week (=7/7) for the original version. It is **1.4** Generations per week (= 7/5) for Delta and **2.0** Generations per week (= 7/3.5) for Omicron. The notation used for Generation speed in this book is **G**.

Reproduction Number or Reproduction Rate R: It is the average number of people infected by a single infected person. The global average value of R at the beginning of the pandemic in early 2020, before preventive measures were enforced, is estimated to be **2.60.** It can be much higher in crowded cities, and lower in the countryside with little inter-human contact. The international notation for Reproduction number is **R**.

If R has a value of 1.0, the number of new infections over any period of time, a week, for example, will stay constant. If the value of R is **below 1.0**, the number of new infections will decline gradually, and the pandemic will disappear ultimately. However, if the value is **above 1.0**, the number of new infections will keep increasing exponentially, as was the case everywhere in early 2020 and is the case in early January 2022 with the Omicron variant spreading fast in many countries around the world.

The Delta variant had pushed R from the painfully achieved value of 1.0 to a catastrophic 2.0 in many countries by mid-2021 because of its increased Generation speed and higher Reproduction rate. By Dec 2021, when Delta was more or less manageable with R around 1.0 to 1.3, Omicron came crashing in with a still higher Generation speed and still higher Reproduction rate than Delta.

* * * *

3   THE MATHEMATICAL PERSPECTIVE OF THE PANDEMIC

From a mathematical perspective, the universal spread of the virus can be best explained in terms of compounding and exponential growth, as described in the sections below.

There are two parallel and mutually complementary processes of compounding and exponential growth that are taking place simultaneously and are feeding the exponential spread of the virus. Metaphorically, those two processes are like what drought and wind are to a wildfire. They are:

1. The **multiplication of the virus particle itself in the human body** that has no immunity or only partial immunity against this virus. These human bodies are akin to dried-up trees in a dense forest in the middle of a drought and where someone has just dropped a burning cigarette.

2. The **multiplication of the number of people infected** through transmission from one infected person to one or more others. It is akin to a strong wind taking the sparks and fire from one burning tree to the neighboring trees.

Let us look at these two processes more closely in the following two sections.

* * * *

4　　MULTIPLICATION OF VIRUS PARTICLES IN THE HUMAN BODY

The information available in the public domain shows that if a Covid-19 virus particle enters a human body that does not generate an immune response, it attaches itself to a human cell, penetrates it, and enters it within about **10 minutes** of coming in physical contact.

Within an average of **12 hours** after infection, the infected cell manufactures an average of about **600 new virus particles** and ejects them out of the cell in a serial process akin to the assembly line of a car manufacturer. Some of those 600 new virus particles float around in the fluidic medium covering the linings of the eyes, nose, mouth, throat, or lungs, and within an average of about **6 hours**, find new cells to penetrate and colonize. Some or most of those 600 virus particles will get destroyed by the body's immune system, depending on how strong the immune system is. However, a part of the 600 virus particles will also get ejected out of the human body through the nose and mouth, some of which may succeed in entering other human bodies and infect them.

The number of new virus particles created from a single parent virus is called the **Viral Yield.** Approximately 600 is the average Viral Yield for the original version of the Corona virus, as reported by some researchers. However, the viral yield may be higher for the Delta and Omicron variants, making them still more infectious.

The **Replication Cycle Time**, i.e., the average time that passes between the infection of a human cell by a virus particle and the sequential infection of another cell in the same human body by its offspring, is about 18 hours (= 12 hours manufacturing time + 6 hours roaming time) for the original version of the virus as reported by some researchers. In other words, it is the time that one virus particle takes to manufacture 600 new ones. This time varies depending on many variables in the human body and can be shorter or longer. The Replication cycle time may be shorter for the Delta and Omicron variants, making them all the more infectious.

For convenience, we will assume that the average replication time is 24 hours for our analysis here.

4.1 INFECTED PERSON WITH PARTIAL IMMUNITY TO CORONA VIRUS

Here, we assume that **50%** of the new virus particles get destroyed by the body's (partial) immune system, **25%** get ejected out of the human body, and the remaining **25%** find a host cell in the same human body and repeat the replication in a chain process. The result will be as follows.

Day 1

New virus particles created: **600** (= 1 x 600).

New virus particles destroyed: **300** (= 50%).

New virus particles ejected out of the human body: **150** (= 25%).

New virus particles staying in the human body and infecting new cells: **150** (= 25%).

Day 2

New virus particles created: **90,000** (= 150 x 600).

New virus particles destroyed: **45,000** (= 50%).

New virus particles ejected out of the human body: **22,500** (= 25%).

New virus particles staying in the human body and infecting new cells: **22,500** (= 25%).

Day 3

New virus particles created: **13.5 million** (= 22,500 x 600).

New virus particles destroyed: **6.8 million** (= 50%).

New virus particles ejected out of the human body: **3.4 million** (= 25%).

New virus particles staying in the human body and infecting new cells: **3.4 million** (= 25%).

Day 4

New virus particles created: **2.0 Billion** (= 3.4 million x 600).

New virus particles destroyed: **1.0 Billion** (= 50%).

New virus particles ejected out of the human body: **0.5 Billion** (= 25%).

New virus particles staying in the human body and infecting new cells: **0.5 Billion** (= 25%).

Day 5

New virus particles created: **300 Billion** (= 0.5 Billion x 600).

New virus particles destroyed: **150 Billion** (= 50%).

New virus particles ejected out of the human body: **75 Billion** (= 25%).

New virus particles staying in the human body and infecting new cells: **75 Billion** (= 25%).

Day 6

New virus particles created: **45.0 Trillion** (= 75 Billion x 600).

New virus particles destroyed: **22.5 Trillion** (= 50%).

New virus particles ejected out of the human body: **11.2 Trillion** (= 25%).

New virus particles staying in the human body and infecting new cells: **11.2 Trillion** (= 25%).

Day 7

New virus particles created: **6,800 Trillion** (= 11.2 Trillion x 600).

New virus particles destroyed: **3,400 Trillion** (= 50%).

New virus particles ejected out of the human body: **1,700 Trillion** (= 25%).

New virus particles staying in the human body and infecting new cells: **1,700 Trillion** (= 25%).

4.2   INFECTED PERSON WITH ZERO IMMUNITY TO CORONA VIRUS

Here, we assume that **none** of the new virus particles get destroyed by the body's dysfunctional immune system, **50%** get ejected from the human body, and the remaining **50%** find a host cell in the same human body and repeat the replication process every time. The result will be as follows.

Day 1

New virus particles created: **600** (= 1 x 600).

New virus particles destroyed: **0**.

New virus particles ejected out of the human body: **300** (= 50%).

New virus particles staying in the human body and infecting new cells: **300** (= 50%).

Day 2

New virus particles created: **180,000** (= 300 x 600).

New virus particles destroyed: **0**.

New virus particles ejected out of the human body: **90,000** (= 50%).

New virus particles staying in the human body and infecting new cells: **90,000** (= 50%).

Day 3

New virus particles created: **54 million** (= 90,00 x 600).

New virus particles destroyed: **0**.

New virus particles ejected out of the human body: **27 million** (= 50%).

New virus particles staying in the human body and infecting new cells: **27 million** (= 50%).

Day 4

New virus particles created: **16 Billion** (= 27 million x 600).

New virus particles destroyed: **0**.

New virus particles ejected out of the human body: **8.0 Billion** (= 50%).

New virus particles staying in the human body and infecting new cells: **8.0 Billion** (= 50%).

Day 5

New virus particles created: **4.8 Trillion** (= 8 Billion x 600).

New virus particles destroyed: **0**.

New virus particles ejected out of the human body: **2.4 Trillion** (= 50%).

New virus particles staying in the human body and infecting new cells: **2.4 Trillion** (= 50%).

Day 6

New virus particles created: **1,440 Trillion** (= 2.4 Trillion x 600).

New virus particles destroyed: **0**.

New virus particles ejected out of the human body: **720 Trillion** (= 50%).

New virus particles staying in the human body and infecting new cells: **720 Trillion** (= 50%).

Day 7

New virus particles created: **432,000 Trillion** (= 720 Trillion x 600).

New virus particles destroyed: **0**.

New virus particles ejected out of the human body: **216,000 Trillion** (= 50%).

New virus particles staying in the human body and infecting new cells: **216,000 Trillion** (= 50%).

4.3   ANALYSIS OF THE NUMBERS AND CONCLUSIONS

What we see here is compounding and the resultant exponential growth at work.

4.3.1   Comparing infected persons with and without immunity

For the person with partial immunity, even with the body's immune system destroying 50% of the newly created virus particles, the number of virus particles in the human body increases by a factor of **150** every 24 hours. This increase factor also applies to the number of virus particles that get ejected and can potentially infect others nearby.

This day-to-day multiplication factor increases from **150** to **300** if the immune system is totally dysfunctional and no virus particle gets destroyed. The consequence is that, at the end of the peak infection period, i.e., at the end of day 7, there will be **128x times more virus particles** in the body as well as in the emissions from that body (128 = 216,000 trillion/1,700 trillion) compared to an infected person with a 50% immunity.

4.3.2   Transmissibility and severity of illness and their correlation to viral load

4.3.2.1   Viral load ratios

The day-to-day **ratio of viral load and infectiousness** between these two infected persons, one with no immunity and the other a partial one, is as below.

Day-1: **2x** more viral load and infectiousness.

Day-2: **4x** more viral load and infectiousness.

Day-3: **8x** more viral load and infectiousness.

Day-4: **16x** more viral load and infectiousness.

Day-5: **32x** more viral load and infectiousness.

Day-6: **64x** more viral load and infectiousness.

Day-7: **128x** more viral load and infectiousness.

4.3.2.2   Correlation of transmissibility and severity of the illness to viral load

> **From the above, we can conclude that the infected person without immunity will be 128 times more infectious at the peak of his infection period than someone with partial (50%) immunity.**

> **Likewise, with 128 times more virus particles in the body and consequently 128 times more tissue cells in the body having been infected and destroyed, he is also likely to be more seriously ill with 128 times more severity.**

4.3.3   Incubation period and its correlation to viral load

4.3.3.1   Viral load numbers

The **viral load** of a person with **partial immunity**, as calculated in <u>section 4.1</u> above, is listed below again for convenience. These are theoretical values, and the multi-trillion values may never be reached due to various biological constraints.

Day-1: **150** virus particles retained as viral load in the human body.

Day-2: **22,500** virus particles retained as viral load in the human body.

Day-3: **3.4 million** virus particles retained as viral load in the human body.

Day-4: **500 million** virus particles retained as viral load in the human body.

Day-5: **75 Billion** virus particles retained as viral load in the human body.

Day-6: **11.2 Trillion** virus particles retained as viral load in the human body.

Day-7: **1,700 Trillion** virus particles retained as viral load in the human body.

4.3.3.2   Correlation of Incubation period to viral load

The end of the incubation period may be the result of the explosive increase of viral load due to exponential growth.

The exponential growth of virus particles in the human body, as is evident from the above list, may also explain why an infected person does not feel sick during the first few days (the incubation period), but the condition deteriorates rapidly after that. **500 million** virus particles in the cells of a human body, as is the case after **4 days**, is of a different order of magnitude than the mere **22,500** after **2 days**. That can make all the difference and explain the sudden illness and rapid worsening of the patient's condition on day-4.

> **The Incubation period, the sudden emergence of illness after that, and the rapid worsening not long after that are clearly the results of the explosive increase of viral load due to compounding and exponential growth.**

4.3.4   Latent period and its correlation to viral load

The exponential growth of virus particles in the human body, as is evident from the above list, may also explain why an infected person does not seem to infect others during the first couple of days after getting infected (the latent period) but suddenly becomes highly infectious after that. For example, the infectiousness of a person ejecting **27 million** virus particles through the mouth and nose on **day-3** is of a different order of magnitude than the infectiousness of the same person on **day-1** when he ejects only **300** virus particles, as the numbers in section 4.2 above show.

> **The latent period and the sudden jump of infectiousness after that are clearly the results of the explosive increase of viral load due to compounding and exponential growth.**

4.3.4.1   The Latent period may not be genuinely latent

The numbers above show that you may be shedding viruses even on the 2nd day after the infection, **even if only in relatively tiny numbers**. Even if tested during the 2nd day, the viral load may be too small to be detected, and you will go home with a negative test result even while you may be shedding the virus, even if in small undetectable quantities. That means, in principle, an infected person may be infectious and may transmit the virus to others just after a single cycle of replication which we have assumed to be 24 hours for the sake of convenience but may be considerably shorter in reality.

Moreover, replication of the Corona virus is **not a batch process but a continuous one**. That means replicated new virus particles may be produced and released from the infected cell within hours of infection and subsequently ejected from the body through the mouth or nose continuously, even if only in tiny numbers at this stage. Reinfecting others is therefore possible even at this early stage, even though our test devices and methods cannot detect them in such low concentrations.

Moreover, it is also more probable that the infected person was infected initially with a thousand or a million virus particles instead of just one particle that we have assumed for our calculations. The numbers in the lists above will then be a thousand or a million times higher, and so also the infectiousness in the early stages.

> **It follows, therefore, that someone who got infected with a million virus particles initially will be highly infectious about 2 days earlier than another person who got infected initially with only a few virus particles.**

The Latent period, defined as the one during which an infected person cannot transmit the virus to others, may be a mirage and not a reality when looked at from a mathematical perspective. All measuring devices have their limitations and minimum thresholds in the real world. The latent period may only mean that the viral load is below this detection threshold and not necessarily absent totally.

Therefore, when looked at from a numerical perspective, some infections may be occurring on the first day itself. On the other hand, a substantial part of the infections may be occurring between days 2 & 5 even before developing any symptoms or even before testing positive, i.e., in the Latent period when infecting others is assumed to be impossible.

In all these cases, the infector cannot know that they are infected and are infectious to some degree.

The popular belief that one becomes infectious only after developing symptoms of illness or testing positive is obviously false. It does not align with the mathematical reality of the number of virus particles in the human body.

> **The Latent period for the Corona virus may be even less than a day when looked at from the mathematical perspective of numbers.**

* * * *

5 SPREAD OF THE VIRUS FROM HUMAN BODY TO HUMAN BODY

As noted in section 3 above, this is the second and parallel process of compounding and exponential growth that is taking place, as seen from a mathematical perspective. This process is akin to a wind that carries sparks and fire from one burning tree to other neighboring trees in a wildfire in a dry, dense forest.

In the sub-sections below, we are taking a quick look at the initial period of the pandemic to illustrate a point. This initial period was contact-traced accurately. The data was analyzed thoroughly by expects as Covid-19 was deadly, small, locally confined, and the zest for knowledge about this new killer was very high.

5.1 THE POWER OF PHYSICAL DISTANCING AND OTHER PREVENTIVE MEASURES

5.1.1 Actual situation worldwide by the end of April 2020, 4.5 months after the outbreak of Covid-19

We assume it started with just one person in Wuhan, China, in mid-Dec 2019. A short **4.5 months later**, by the end of April 2020, there were about **3.9 million** infections worldwide.

The **average Generation time**, i.e., the average period between getting infected and infecting others, was about **7 days** for the original version, as was concluded by WHO and most scientists in early 2020. Therefore, based on the above numbers, it can be calculated that, on average, one infected person must have passed it on to **2.15** others.

In just **19 steps** or Generations or cycles of compounding at a growth rate of only **2.15x infections per step**, the virus had spread to about **3.9 million people.**

The involved number of infections per step are given in Table 1 and Figure 1 below to make it easier for the reader to grasp.

By the end of April 2020, the "**Reproduction Number**", i.e., the average number of people to whom one infected person transmits the virus, had probably dropped to **below 1.0** in some countries. It meant that the exponential growth had been stopped, and the number of newly infected people would keep on falling, even if only slowly and gradually.

From a Reproduction number of **6.0** in the beginning in Wuhan, as explained in section 5.1.2 below, to less than **1.0** in 19 weeks in China and some other countries is an achievement that was only possible with the drastic lockdowns, social distancing, and other preventive measures implemented vigorously in those countries.

5.1.2   Actual situation in the first six weeks in Wuhan

The average position, as shown in Table 1 and Figure 1, is what we got after implementing all the social distancing and lockdown measures worldwide. However, there were no such containment measures in Wuhan in the beginning. Based on the total number of infections in Wuhan in the first 1.5 months, it has been estimated that, on average, one infected person might have passed on the virus to **6** others, resulting in about **56,000 infections**. That happened in only **6 steps of 6 transmissions each** because of the exponential effect of compounding. In a crowded megacity like Wuhan, the infection rate, expressed as Reproduction number, will be higher than in other thinner populated areas.

5.1.3   What if there were no lockdowns, social distancing, and other preventive measures?

See Table 2 for the catastrophic situation if there were no preventive measures like lockdowns and social distancing worldwide.

It was estimated by WHO and other agencies in early 2020 that, if left uncontained through lockdowns and quarantine measures, the average Reproduction rate would be approximately **2.6** at an average transmission cycle time of **7 days**. Therefore, if we calculate the compounding effect based on these figures, the number of infections worldwide would have been about **125 million** by the end of April 2020 instead of the actual **3.9 million** reached.

That means there would have been a 32-fold increase in infections and deaths by April 2020 without strict containment measures worldwide.

5.1.4   Conclusions

In the first 4.5 months of the Covid-19 pandemic, i.e., from mid-Dec 2019 till the end of April 2020, we managed to contain the human toll of the virus to 3% of the potential toll, preventing 97% of the potential toll of infections and deaths through effective preventive measures.

In theory, without the preventive measures, most of the world population would have been infected by the end of May 2020, hardly half a year from the outbreak's start.

I am convinced that I am alive today thanks to the effective preventive measures imposed by the government of my country (The Netherlands). So also, probably a considerable percentage of those protesting today violently against the preventive measures are alive and well today thanks to the very same preventive measures against which they are agitating.

Luckily, scientists and statisticians with knowledge of the effects of compounding had stepped forward to persuade reluctant governments to enforce lockdowns, social distancing, and many other preventive measures despite the violent protests by a small minority.

Average progression of Covid-19 Infections in 4.5 months with the benefits of all preventive measures			
Reproduction Number per infected person per period of 7 days			2.15
Period	Week ending on	Newly Infected people	Total infected people
0	16-Dec-19	1	1
1	23-Dec-19	2	3
2	30-Dec-19	5	8
3	06-Jan-20	10	18
4	13-Jan-20	21	39
5	20-Jan-20	46	85
6	27-Jan-20	99	184
7	03-Feb-20	212	396
8	10-Feb-20	457	853
9	17-Feb-20	982	1,834
10	24-Feb-20	2,110	3,945
11	02-Mar-20	4,538	8,482
12	09-Mar-20	9,756	18,238
13	16-Mar-20	20,975	39,213
14	23-Mar-20	45,096	84,309
15	30-Mar-20	96,956	181,266
16	06-Apr-20	208,456	389,722
17	13-Apr-20	448,181	837,903
18	20-Apr-20	963,590	1,801,493
19	27-Apr-20	2,071,718	3,873,212

Table 1: Average progression of Covid-19 infections worldwide in 4.5 months, including the effects of all preventive measures.

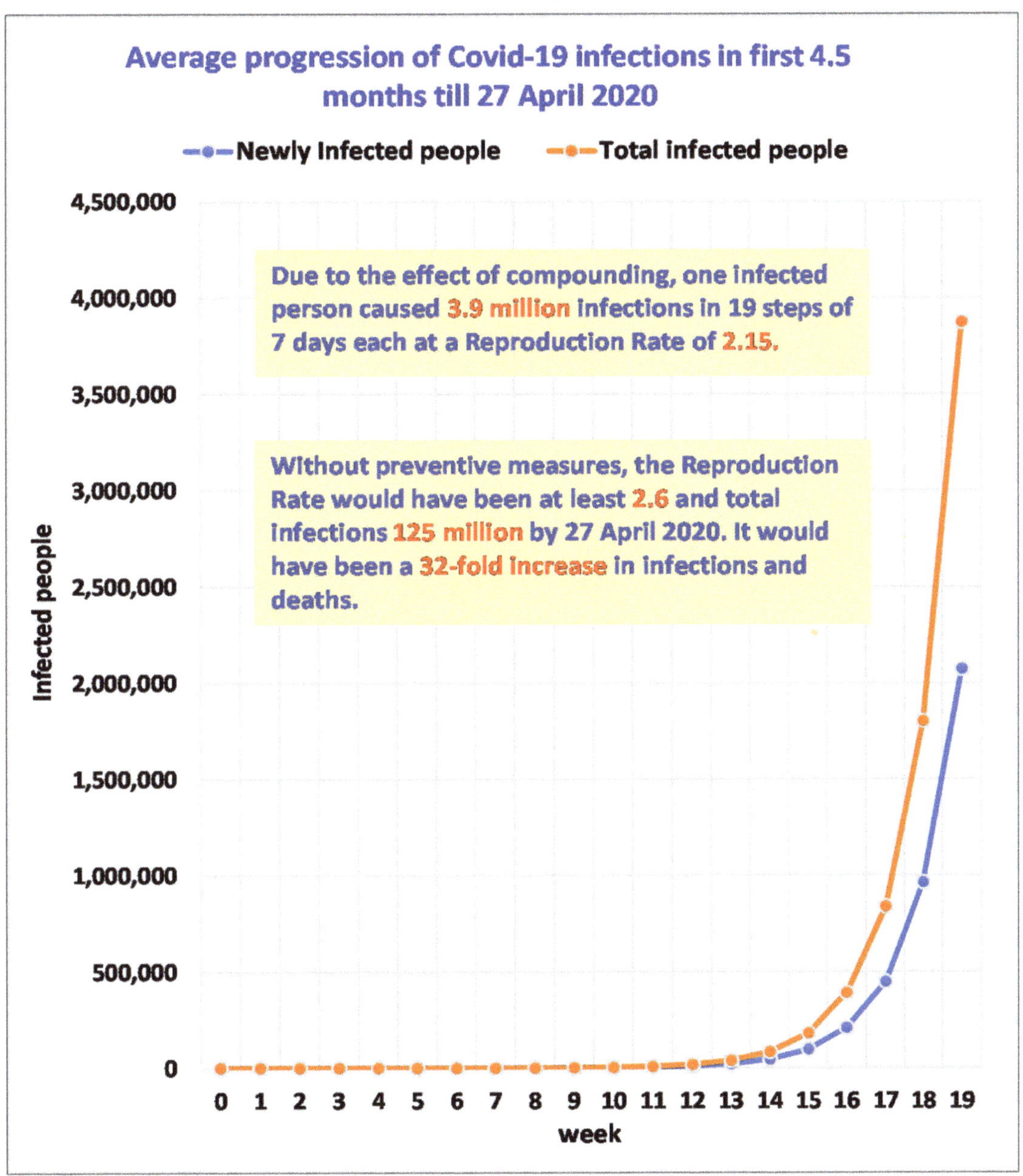

Figure 1: Average progression of Covid-19 infections worldwide in the first 4.5 months, including the effects of all preventive measures.

All values in this Figure are taken from Table 1

Average progression of Covid-19 Infections in 4.5 months without lockdowns and social distancing			
Reproduction Number per infected person per period of 7 days			2.60
Period	Week ending on	Newly Infected people	Total infected people
0	16-Dec-19	1	1
1	23-Dec-19	3	4
2	30-Dec-19	7	10
3	06-Jan-20	18	28
4	13-Jan-20	46	74
5	20-Jan-20	119	192
6	27-Jan-20	309	501
7	03-Feb-20	803	1,305
8	10-Feb-20	2,088	3,393
9	17-Feb-20	5,430	8,822
10	24-Feb-20	14,117	22,939
11	02-Mar-20	36,703	59,642
12	09-Mar-20	95,429	155,071
13	16-Mar-20	248,115	403,187
14	23-Mar-20	645,100	1,048,286
15	30-Mar-20	1,677,259	2,725,546
16	06-Apr-20	4,360,874	7,086,420
17	13-Apr-20	11,338,273	18,424,693
18	20-Apr-20	29,479,510	47,904,203
19	27-Apr-20	76,646,727	124,550,930

Table 2: Average progression of Covid-19 infections worldwide in 4.5 months if there were not any preventive measures.

5.2   ACTUAL SITUATION WORLDWIDE BY 1 JANUARY 2022, TWO YEARS AFTER THE OUTBREAK OF COVID-19

At the time of this update, 10 January 2022, the latest data from WHO shows the following:

Total infections worldwide till 31 December 2021: **285 million.**

12 months earlier, on 31 December 2020, this figure was **84 million.** That is an increase by a factor of **3.4** (= 285/ 84) or an increase by 201 million (= 285 – 84) in 12 months. That amounts to a month-on-month increase of **10.7%** per month in the year 2021. Due to the effect of compounding, the 10.7% per month grew to 3.4-fold in 12 months.

The total number of deaths worldwide officially reported till 31 December 2021 is **5.4 million.** One year earlier, on 31 December 2020, this cumulative figure was **1.9 million.** That is an increase by a factor of **2.8** (= 5.4/ 1.9), but lower than the 3.4-fold increase in infections. The cumulative mortality rate decreased from **2.3%** (= 1.9/84) in 2020 to **1.9%** (= 5.4/285) in 2021.

If we consider the year 2021 individually, the number of infections was 201 million and deaths 3.5 million. That is a mortality rate of **1.75%.** By contrast, during the peak of the first wave in early 2020, with hospitals overwhelmed in many countries and Oxygen in short supply, the mortality rate was about **5.0%.**

Daily new infections worldwide on 30 December 2021 was **1.4 million** (per day). One year ago, at the end of Dec 2020, this figure was considerably lower, with only **0.4 million** new infections in a day. It is an increase by a **factor of 3.5** (= 1.4/ 0.4).

5.3   HOW MANY LIVES WERE SAVED BY LOCKDOWNS AND OTHER PREVENTIVE MEASURES?

If we look at the numbers in section 5.2 above, **5.4** million of the **285** million infected people died till 31 December 2021. So that is a mortality rate of about **1.9%** (= 5.4/ 285).

During the first wave of the virus in 2020, the death toll was about **5%** worldwide, partly because hospitals were overwhelmed in many countries with a shortage of even basic necessities such as Oxygen.

As noted in section 5.1.4 above, most of the world population would have been infected by mid-2020 if the lockdowns and other preventive measures were not implemented rigorously in many countries.

The world has a population of 7.8 Billion, of which **5.2 Billion** are above 20 years of age. If all of them got infected and a tsunami of infections had rolled over the world in 2020, hospitals everywhere would have been totally overwhelmed with no bed, no staff, and no equipment, and most of the severely ill people would have died in the streets, or at best, at home. Moreover, without the IC and other medical support, the 5% mortality rate of the first wave would have gone still higher.

If we assume a 5% mortality rate even in such an apocalyptic situation, the death toll would have been **260 million** (= 5% of 5.2 Billion). Even if we assume the potential mortality to be half of it, it is still **130 million** lives saved. If we take the mortality rate of the Spanish Flu of 1918-20 as a reference, we would have lost about **220 million** lives (2.8% of the population). However, we avoided it by implementing lockdowns and other preventive measures.

With all the lockdowns and other preventive measures, we achieved the following.

- Instead of 5.2 Billion, we managed to limit the number of infections to 285 million. That is a **reduction of 94.5% or an 18-fold reduction**.

- This hugely reduced number of infections could be stretched over **2 years** instead of **6 months,** ensuring that hospitals were not overwhelmed and that most patients could get the needed medical attention.

- We bought time to develop vaccines and immunize a majority of the world population, in the meantime shielding about 94.5% of the infectible population from getting infected.

> - **Above all, we saved at least 130 million lives by enduring lockdowns and other restrictive measures. That means at least half of humanity was spared of potential intense grief at the loss of a dear one. We managed to limit the loss of lives to 5.4 million, preventing 96% of the possible loss of lives.**

It is a collective sacrifice and achievement that we all can be proud of.

* * * *

6   DELTA VARIANT

By Sept 2021, it was established by the scientific community that the Delta variant is substantially more catastrophic than the original version due to **two fundamental changes** in how it infects humans.

1. The average Generation time decreased from **7 days** for the original version to **5 days** for Delta. That means, on average, an infected person infects another person in about 5 days instead of 7 before. That means the **Generation speed** will be **1.40 Generations per week** (= 7/5) for Delta while it is 1.00 for the original version (= 7/7). The consequence is that there will be **40% more Generation cycles or transmission cycles** in a week, or any period for that matter, than was the case with the original version.

2. Adding further to the increased maliciousness of Delta is the fact that Delta is **2x times as infectious** as the original version. On average, one infected person passes on the virus to **2x times** as many people as was the case with the original version of the virus. In mathematical terms, the **Reproduction number R is 2x times higher**. For example, if R was 1.2 earlier, it is 2.4 for Delta.

Experts attribute the increased and compounded maliciousness of the Delta variant to mutations that have resulted in the virus having considerably **more spikes** capable of attaching to and penetrating a human cell than the original version of the virus.

As reported by the scientific community, the fact that there are about **1,000x times more virus particles** in the respiratory tracts of people infected with Delta than with the original version may also be another significant contributing factor to the doubling of the Reproduction number and the shortened Generation time.

The two behavioral changes mentioned above, namely the **40%** higher Generation speed and the **doubled** Reproduction rate, can be understood and explained best through the mathematics of compounding, as is done throughout the rest of this book.

6.1   DELTA: THE EFFECT OF DOUBLING OF REPRODUCTION NUMBER R

We will cover this topic in detail in section 8 below.

See section 8.1 for the actual number of infections for various R values.

See section 8.3.1 to see by which factor the weekly infection rates will increase due to the **doubling** of R.

The effects of doubling the Reproduction number have already been incorporated in the **Corona Tables** presented in section 10 below.

6.2   DELTA: THE EFFECT OF DECREASE OF GENERATION TIME FROM 7 DAYS TO 5 DAYS, OR INCREASE OF GENERATION SPEED WITH 40%

Please see section 7.2 below, which covers this topic that is common to both Delta and Omicron.

* * * *

7   OMICRON VARIANT

As of the beginning of 2022, it has been established by the scientific community that the Omicron variant is substantially more infectious than the original version or the Delta variant. As was also the case with Delta, the increased infectiousness may be due to **two fundamental changes** in how it infects humans.

1. The average Generation time has decreased further to about **3.5** days from the **5** days for Delta and **7** days for the original version. That means the **Generation speed** of Omicron is **2.0 Generations per week** (= 7/3.5) while it is **1.40 for Delta** and **1.0 for the original version**. Therefore, it follows that the Generation speed of Omicron is **43%** (= 1.5/3.5) higher than that of Delta and 100% higher than that of the original version.

2. Adding further to the increased maliciousness is the fact that Omicron is probably **3x times as infectious** as the original version, while Delta was only **2x** times as infectious as the original version. That means, on average, one infected person passes on the virus to 3x times as many people as was the case with the original version. In mathematical terms, the **Reproduction number R is 3x times higher**. For example, if R was 1.2 with the original version, it is 2.4 for Delta and 3.6 for Omicron. That means, on average, one person infected with Omicron transmits the virus to 3.6 others instead of 1.2 with the original version and 2.4 with Delta. It follows from the above that the Reproduction number of Omicron is **50% higher than that of Delta**, which is to say it is **1.50x** times higher.

Experts attribute the aggravated and compounded infectiousness of Omicron to about 30 mutations with respect to the Delta variant.

The two behavioral changes mentioned above, namely the **100%** higher Generation speed and the **tripled** Reproduction rate compared to the original version, can be understood and explained best through the mathematics of compounding. It is so because it is the compounding of these two mutually complementary changes that is fueling the accelerated spread of Omicron around the world, as explained throughout the rest of this book.

7.1   OMICRON: THE EFFECT OF THE TRIPLING OF REPRODUCTION NUMBER R

We will cover this topic in detail in section 8 below.

See section 8.1 for the actual number of infections for various R values.

See section 8.3.2 to see by which factor the weekly infection rates will increase due to the **tripling** of R.

The effects of the tripling of the Reproduction number have already been incorporated in the **Corona Tables** presented in section 10 below.

7.2   OMICRON: THE EFFECT OF DECREASE OF GENERATION TIME FROM 7 DAYS TO 3.5 DAYS, OR INCREASE OF GENERATION SPEED WITH 100%

The mathematics of the increase of Generation speed is too complex for the lay reader, and therefore the mathematical details are not included in this book. However, as discussed in section 9 below, its effect can be read indirectly from the Corona Tables provided in section 10 and Appendix-A below.

For the more math-savvy reader, the share of Generation speed on the growth rate of infections can be calculated using the formula R^G which will give the weekly growth rate of infections as explained in section 11 below.

In addition, section 12 shows, with examples, how much the individual share of Generation speed will be in the growth rate of weekly infections and how that relates to the share of Reproduction number R.

> **As shown in section 12, the shock wave of infections that we have been witnessing lately with Omicron, and to a lesser extent with Delta earlier, have been caused mainly by the increased Generation speed of those two variants.**

* * * *

8   THE EFFECT OF REPRODUCTION NUMBER R ON INFECTION RATES

Assuming that the Generation speed is **1.0 generation per week,** as was the case with the original version of the virus, let us first calculate the actual number of weekly new infections if one person gets infected. Then let us see how much, or by which factor, the existing infections will increase if the Reproduction number jumps to a higher value.

8.1   THE ACTUAL NUMBER OF INFECTIONS

8.1.1   Reproduction number 1.0

New infections in week-1: **1**

New infections in week-2: 1^2 = **1**

New infections in week-3: 1^3 = **1**

New infections in week-4: 1^4 = **1**

New infections in week-5: 1^5 = **1**

New infections in week-10: 1^{10} = **1**

8.1.2   Reproduction number 1.5

New infections in week-1: **1.5**

New infections in week-2: 1.5^2 = **2.3**

New infections in week-3: 1.5^3 = **3.4**

New infections in week-4: 1.5^4 = **5.1**

New infections in week-5: 1.5^5 = **7.6**

New infections in week-10: 1.5^{10} = **57.7**

8.1.3 Reproduction number 2.0

New infections in week-1: **2**

New infections in week-2: 2^2 = **4**

New infections in week-3: 2^3 = **8**

New infections in week-4: 2^4 = **16**

New infections in week-5: 2^5 = **32**

New infections in week-10: 2^{10} = **1,024**

8.1.4 Reproduction number 3.0

New infections in week-1: **3**

New infections in week-2: 3^2 = **9**

New infections in week-3: 3^3 = **27**

New infections in week-4: 3^4 = **81**

New infections in week-5: 3^5 = **243**

New infections in week-10: 3^{10} = **59,049**

8.1.5 Reproduction number 4.0

New infections in week-1: **4**

New infections in week-2: 4^2 = **16**

New infections in week-3: 4^3 = **64**

New infections in week-4: 4^4 = **256**

New infections in week-5: 4^5 = **1,024**

New infections in week-10: 4^{10} = **1,048,576**

8.2 ANALYSIS OF THE ACTUAL NUMBER OF INFECTIONS

Assuming that the Generation speed is **1.0 generation per week**, and the Reproduction number is **1.0**, the weekly new infections will be limited to a steady 1.0 infection every week.

If the Reproduction number is **2.0**, the weekly new infections will increase exponentially by a factor of 2.0 every week, reaching **1,024** new infections in **week-10**.

If the Reproduction number is **4.0**, the weekly new infections will increase exponentially by a factor of 4.0 every week, reaching **more than a million** new infections in **week-10.**

It is evident from the above numbers that **the higher the Reproduction number, the steeper the increase of weekly new infections.**

> **The initial value of Reproduction number R and the number of weeks passed are two of the three crucial factors determining the growth in the number of new infections. The third, and almost always the most influential player in the case of Omicron, is Generation time which we will discuss in detail later in this book.**

8.3 THE GROWTH FACTOR OF INFECTIONS IF REPRODUCTION NUMBER R INCREASES

We have already seen the effect of Reproduction number on the **actual number** of infections in section 8.1 above. But as we will be dealing with doubling and tripling of Reproduction numbers in the following sections, we will discuss here **how much, or by which factor**, the actual infections will increase due to the doubling or tripling of the Reproduction number or increasing it by a factor 1.5.

8.3.1   If Reproduction Number R doubles from 1R to 2R

We are looking at the doubling of R because, as we have seen in section 6 above, when **Delta** displaces the original version, the value of R will double due to the higher infectiousness of Delta.

The Reproduction number will also double or climb even higher if existing social restrictions are lifted too drastically.

The **factor** by which the **weekly new infections** will increase solely because the Reproduction number doubles from **1R to 2R** is as below.

Week-1:

Original Infection rate: 1R

New infection rate: 2R

Ratio of increase: 2R/1R = 2^1 = **2.0**

Week-2:

Original Infection rate: 1R x 1R = $1R^2$

New infection rate: 2R x 2R = $4R^2$

Ratio of increase: $4R^2/1R^2$ = 2^2 = **4.0**

Week-5:

Original Infection rate: 1R x 1R x 1R x 1R x 1R = $1R^5$

New infection rate: 2R x 2R x 2R x 2R x 2R = $32R^5$

Ratio of increase: $32R^5/1R^5$ = 2^5 = **32**

Similarly, we also get the following.

Week-9: 2^9 = **512x** times higher infections than infections without the doubling of R.

Week-13: 2^{13} = **8,192x** times higher infections than infections without the doubling of R.

Week-N: 2^N times higher infections in week-N than infections without the doubling of R.

Week-4.33 (last week of month-1): $2^{4.33}$ = **20.2x** times higher weekly infections than infections without the doubling of R.

Week-8.67 (last week of month-2): $2^{8.67}$ = **406x** times higher weekly infections than infections without the doubling of R.

Week-13 (last week of month-3): 2^{13} = **8,192x** times higher weekly infections than infections without the doubling of R.

8.3.2   If Reproduction Number R triples from 1R to 3R

We are looking at the tripling of R because, as we have seen in section 7 above, when **Omicron** displaces the original version, the value of R will triple due to the higher infectiousness of Omicron.

The method of calculation is the same as in section 8.3.1 above.

The **factor** by which the **weekly new infections** will increase solely because the Reproduction number triples from **1R to 3R** is as below.

Week 1: **3x** times higher infections than the infections without the tripling of R.

Week-2: 3^2 times = **9x** times higher infections than infections without the tripling of R.

Week-5: 3^5 times = **243x** times higher infections than infections without the tripling of R.

Week-9: 3^9 times = **19,683x** times higher infections than infections without the tripling of R.

Week-13: 3^{13} times = **1.6 million** times higher infections than infections without the tripling of R.

Week-4.33 (last week of month-1): $3^{4.33}$ = **117x** times higher weekly infections than infections without the tripling of R.

Week-8.67 (last week of month-2): $3^{8.67}$ = **13,647x** times higher weekly infections than infections without the tripling of R.

Week-13 (last week of month-3): 3^{13} = **1.6 million** times higher weekly infections than infections without the tripling of R.

8.3.3 If Reproduction Number R increases from 1R to 1.5R

We are looking at the increase of R by a factor of 1.5 because, as we have seen in <u>section 7</u> above, when **Omicron** displaces **Delta**, the value of R will increase by 50% due to the higher infectiousness of Omicron.

The **factor** by which the **weekly new infections** will increase because the Reproduction number increases from **1R to 1.5R** is as below.

Week 1: **1.5x** times higher infections than infections without the 50% increase of R.

Week-2: 1.5^{2} times = **2.25x** times higher infections than infections without the 50% increase of R.

Week-5: 1.5^{5} times = **7.6x** times higher infections than infections without the 50% increase of R.

Week-9: 1.5^{9} times = **38x** times higher infections than infections without the 50% increase of R.

Week-13: 1.5^{13} times = **195x** times higher infections than infections without the 50% increase of R.

Week-4.33 (last week of month-1): $1.5^{4.33}$ = **5.8x** times higher weekly infections than infections without the 50% increase of R.

Week-8.67 (last week of month-2): $1.5^{8.67}$ = **34x** times higher weekly infections than infections without the 50% increase of R.

Week-13 (last week of month-3): 1.5^{13} = **195x** times higher weekly infections than infections without the 50% increase of R.

8.4   ANALYSIS OF THE GROWTH FACTOR OF INFECTIONS DUE TO THE INCREASE OF REPRODUCTION NUMBER

The above numbers are **GROWTH FACTORS** showing how much the infections will multiply solely due to the increase of R.

The GROWTH FACTORS are independent of the Reproduction number R's initial value. Therefore, they apply equally to any initial value of R.

For example, as seen in section 8.3.1, if the initial value of R is **1.5** and it doubles to **3.0**, there will be a **32-fold** increase in infections in week-5 compared to the infections without the doubling. That means the actual number of infections will increase from **7.6** as seen in section 8.1.2 to **243** as seen in section 8.1.4, a **32-fold** increase.

> **As is evident from the numbers in section 8.1 and section 8.3 above, the ACTUAL NUMBER of weekly new infections is influenced tremendously by the initial value of R, the factor by which it increased due to a new variant or a change in social behavior, and the time that has elapsed since the increase of Reproduction number.**

* * * *

9   THE EFFECT OF GENERATION SPEED G ON INFECTION RATES

As we have already seen in section 6 and section 7 above, the Generation time decreases from 7 days for the original version to **5** days for **Delta** and **3.5** days for **Omicron**. Further details are given in the corresponding sections below.

Delta: A reduction of Generation time from **7** days to **5** days for Delta means, on average, an infected person infects another person in about 5 days instead of 7 before. That means the **Generation speed** will be **1.40 Generations per week** (= 7/5) for Delta while it is 1.00 for the original version (= 7/7). The consequence is that there will be **40% more Generation cycles or transmission cycles** in a week, or any period of time for that matter, than was the case with the original version.

Omicron: The decrease of Generation time from **7** days to **3.5** days for Omicron means an infected person infects another person in about 3.5 days instead of 7 before. That means the **Generation speed** will be **2.0 Generations per week** (= 7/3.5) for Omicron. The consequence is that there will be **100% more Generation cycles or transmission cycles** in a week, or any period of time for that matter, than was the case with the original version.

Omicron: It follows from the above that the Generation speed of Omicron is **43%** (= 1.5/3.5) higher than that of Delta, while it is 100% higher than that of the original version.

Please note that we are talking here about 40% or 100% or 43% more **transmission cycles** and *not* **the number of transmissions**.

Even if everything else remains unchanged, including the Reproduction number, social distancing, and other preventive measures, it is evident that, with a shortened Generation time of 5 or 3.5 days, there will be more infections in a 7-day period (a week) than was the case with the original Generation time of 7 days. How much more the increase of infections will be, depends on the prevailing Reproduction number R before Delta or Omicron displaces the older variant.

The calculations involved with Generation Time's effect on infection rates are somewhat complex because the Reproduction number and the time factor also come into play. Therefore, instead of going into mathematical details in this book, you are given the formulas used and the final results of the calculations in a series of tables dubbed **Corona Tables**.

The effect of the increased Generation speed of Delta or Omicron on the growth rate of infections can be obtained using any of the following methods explained more in detail in the corresponding sections that follow.

1. The **Corona Growth Code**, the formula which gives the growth factor for weekly new infections, is presented and explained in section 11 below. In essence, for those who are a bit handy with calculations, this formula is all that is needed to calculate the rate of weekly infections with any variant with any Reproduction number in any week in the future. The basic formula for the growth rate of weekly infections is R^G, in which R is the Reproduction number and G is the Generation speed in Generations per week.

2. An extension of the above formula, R^{GN}, will give directly by which factor the weekly infections would increase in week N further down the road. For example, for the growth factor of infections 4 weeks from now, the value of N will be 4. This formula is also explained further in section 11. The relative share of G compared to R in the total growth factor of infections can be obtained by substituting G with 1.0 in the formula and comparing the results.

3. The **Corona Tables** are presented in section 10 below. The effects of the increase of Generation speed on weekly infection rates are incorporated in the **Corona Tables** for both Delta and Omicron, and they cover a range of Reproduction numbers and time periods. The tables contain more helpful information than the weekly growth rates obtained using the formulas.

4. Section 12 below shows how much the individual share of Generation speed will be in the total growth rate of weekly infections and how that relates to the share of Reproduction number R.

You will discover that the increased speed of transmissions, especially the doubled speed of Omicron, has enormous consequences for the number of infections, as you will see throughout the rest of this book.

* * * *

10   CORONA TABLES

As mentioned earlier, some of the calculations involved with the growth rate of Covid-19 infections are rather complex and will therefore be of little use to a lay reader to include them here. However, considering the supreme relevance and currency of the topic, all the relevant results of such calculations have been taken up in tables, the **Corona Tables,** and are included in this book. They cover a wide range of parameters, as detailed below.

10.1   THE 4 TYPES OF CORONA TABLES

The Corona Tables comprise of the following 4 types.

10.1.1   Corona Tables, Full version

It consists of 7 pages, with each page covering a range of Reproduction numbers as shown below. Because it occupies 7 pages, only page-1 is shown in the body of this book as Table 3, and the complete table is positioned towards the back end of this book. You can go to the desired page using the hyperlinks here.

Corona Table Page-1: Reproduction numbers: 0.70, 0.80, 0.90, 0.95, 1.00, 1.05, 1.10, 1.15, 1.20, 1.25.

Corona Table Page-2: Reproduction numbers: 1.30, 1.40, 1.50, 1.60, 1.70, 1.80, 1.90, 2.00.

Corona Table Page-3: Reproduction numbers: 2.10, 2.20, 2.30, 2.40, 2.50, 2.60, 2.70.

Corona Table Page-4: Reproduction numbers: 2.80, 2.90, 3.00, 3.20, 3.40, 3.50, 3.60.

Corona Table Page-5: Reproduction numbers: 3.80, 4.00, 4.20, 4.40, 4.50, 4.60, 4.80.

Corona Table Page-6: Reproduction numbers: 5.00, 5.50, 6.00, 6.50, 7.00, 7.50.

Corona Table Page-7: Reproduction numbers: 8.00, 8.50, 9.00, 9.50, 10.00.

10.1.2   Corona Table, Condensed version

It is a one-page table covering the most relevant Reproduction numbers. The Reproduction numbers are: 1.00, 1.20, 1.50, 1.80, 2.00, 2.40, 3.00, 3.60, 4.00, 4.50. Go to Table 4 for the Condensed version.

10.1.3   Corona Table, Jump version

The same as the Condensed version, but with color codes corresponding to the jump from one variant to another. Go to Table 5 for the Jump version.

10.1.4   Corona Table, Future version

The same as the Condensed version, but with Reproduction numbers 1.80, 2.40 & 3.60 omitted due to size constraints and the original version of the virus substituted by a **hypothetical future version** with a shorter Generation time of only **2.5 days** as against Omicron's 3.5 days. Go to Table 6 for the Future version.

10.2   WHAT EACH CORONA TABLE SHOWS

For ease of reference, see Table 4, the Condensed version of the Corona table.

The table is developed using only information available in the public domain. It contains the mathematically expected growth rates of Covid-19 infections with Omicron, Delta, and the original version of the virus. The table shows the actual number of NEW (not cumulative) infections per week and other relevant data if one person gets infected.

As you can see, each table contains three vertically stapled blocks. The top block covers the **original version** of the virus, the middle block covers **Delta**, and the bottom block covers **Omicron.**

All Corona Tables contain the theoretical weekly growth rates of infections and other relevant information as listed below.

1. The **number of weekly new infections** for weeks 1, 2, 3 & 4 that originate from one single infected person.

2. The **number of weekly new infections** for the last weeks of **first, second, and third months** that originate from one infected person.

3. The **Growth Factor** by which **weekly new infections** increase week-to-week and month-to-month.

4. The **day-to-day increase** of new infections, in %.

5. The **doubling time** of new infections in days & hours.

6. If the Reproduction number **R is below 1.0**, the table shows the time, in days and hours, that it will take for the weekly new infections to decrease to **half** the current level.

All tables show the weekly GROWTH RATES of infections, i.e., if ONE SINGLE PERSON gets infected with a particular variant and spreads it further, how it will grow further in the community.

If there are 1,000 infected people in a city at any given time, you only need to multiply the number in the table by 1,000 to get the total number of new infections in any week down the road.

10.3   ASSUMPTIONS MADE FOR THE CORONA TABLES

The tables are calculated based on the following assumptions.

The Generation Time: **7 days** for the original version, **5 days** for Delta, and **3.5 days** for Omicron. That means there will be 1.0 infection cycles per week for the original version, 1.4 infection cycles per week for Delta, and 2.0 infection cycles per week for Omicron.

Each column in the table shows the infection rates if the community's social behavior and immunization level remain unchanged. However, suppose changes are effected to any of these parameters either as part of efforts to curb the spread of the virus or due to the changes in social behavior. In that case, you will need to jump to another column in the table with a correspondingly lower or higher Reproduction number.

CORONA TABLE									Page 1
THEORETICAL WEEKLY NEW COVID-19 INFECTIONS ORIGINATING FROM ONE INFECTED PERSON									
ORIGINAL version	Generation time, days -->		7.0		Generation speed (G), Gen/ week -->				1.00
Reproduction number (R) >	0.70	0.80	0.90	0.95	1.00	1.05	1.10	1.15	1.20	1.25
Week-1	0.70	0.80	0.90	0.95	1.00	1.05	1.10	1.15	1.20	1.25
Week-2	0.49	0.64	0.81	0.90	1.00	1.10	1.21	1.32	1.44	1.56
Week-3	0.34	0.51	0.73	0.86	1.00	1.16	1.33	1.52	1.73	1.95
Week-4	0.24	0.41	0.66	0.81	1.00	1.22	1.46	1.75	2.07	2.44
Last week of Month-1	0.21	0.38	0.63	0.80	1.00	1.24	1.51	1.83	2.20	2.63
Last week of Month-2	0.05	0.14	0.40	0.64	1.00	1.5	2.3	3.4	4.9	6.9
Last week of Month-3	0.01	0.05	0.25	0.51	1.00	1.9	3.5	6.2	10.7	18.2
Week-to-week growth factor	0.70	0.80	0.90	0.95	1.00	1.05	1.10	1.15	1.20	1.25
Month-to-month growth factor	0.21	0.38	0.63	0.80	1.00	1.24	1.51	1.83	2.20	2.63
Day-to-day growth, %	-5.0%	-3.1%	-1.5%	-0.7%	0.0%	0.7%	1.4%	2.0%	2.6%	3.2%
Doubling/ halving time, days	-13.6	-21.7	-46.1	-94.6	Infinity	99.4	50.9	34.7	26.6	21.7
Doubling/ halving time, hours	-326	-522	-1,105	-2,270	Infinity	2,387	1,222	833	639	522
DELTA variant	Generation time, days -->		5.0		Generation speed (G), Gen/ week -->				1.40
Reproduction number (R) >	0.70	0.80	0.90	0.95	1.00	1.05	1.10	1.15	1.20	1.25
Week-1	0.92	1.07	1.23	1.32	1.40	1.48	1.57	1.66	1.74	1.83
Week-2	0.56	0.79	1.07	1.23	1.40	1.59	1.79	2.02	2.25	2.51
Week-3	0.34	0.57	0.92	1.14	1.40	1.70	2.05	2.45	2.91	3.42
Week-4	0.21	0.42	0.79	1.06	1.40	1.82	2.34	2.98	3.75	4.68
Last week of Month-1	0.17	0.38	0.75	1.04	1.40	1.86	2.45	3.18	4.09	5.19
Last week of Month-2	0.02	0.10	0.40	0.76	1.40	2.5	4.4	7.4	12.3	20.1
Last week of Month-3	0.00	0.03	0.21	0.56	1.40	3.4	7.8	17.3	37.3	77.9
Week-to-week growth factor	0.61	0.73	0.86	0.93	1.00	1.07	1.14	1.22	1.29	1.37
Month-to-month growth factor	0.11	0.26	0.53	0.73	1.00	1.34	1.78	2.33	3.02	3.87
Day-to-day growth, %	-6.9%	-4.4%	-2.1%	-1.0%	0.0%	1.0%	1.9%	2.8%	3.7%	4.6%
Doubling/ halving time, days	-9.7	-15.5	-32.9	-67.6	Infinity	71.0	36.4	24.8	19.0	15.5
Doubling/ halving time, hours	-233	-373	-789	-1,622	Infinity	1,705	873	595	456	373
OMICRON variant	Generation time, days -->		3.5		Generation speed (G), Gen/ week -->				2.00
Reproduction number (R) >	0.70	0.80	0.90	0.95	1.00	1.05	1.10	1.15	1.20	1.25
Week-1	1.19	1.44	1.71	1.85	2.00	2.15	2.31	2.47	2.64	2.81
Week-2	0.58	0.92	1.39	1.67	2.00	2.37	2.80	3.27	3.80	4.39
Week-3	0.29	0.59	1.12	1.51	2.00	2.62	3.38	4.32	5.47	6.87
Week-4	0.14	0.38	0.91	1.36	2.00	2.88	4.09	5.72	7.88	10.73
Last week of Month-1	0.11	0.33	0.85	1.32	2.00	2.98	4.36	6.28	8.90	12.45
Last week of Month-2	0.01	0.05	0.34	0.84	2.00	4.5	10	21	43	86
Last week of Month-3	0.00	0.01	0.14	0.54	2.00	6.9	23	71	210	596
Week-to-week growth factor	0.49	0.64	0.81	0.90	1.00	1.10	1.21	1.32	1.44	1.56
Month-to-month growth factor	0.05	0.14	0.40	0.64	1.00	1.53	2.28	3.36	4.86	6.92
Day-to-day growth, %	-9.7%	-6.2%	-3.0%	-1.5%	0.0%	1.4%	2.8%	4.1%	5.3%	6.6%
Doubling/ halving time, days	-6.8	-10.9	-23.0	-47.3	Infinity	49.7	25.5	17.4	13.3	10.9
Doubling/ halving time, hours	-163	-261	-553	-1,135	Infinity	1,193	611	417	319	261

Table 3: Corona Table, page 1: Theoretical WEEKLY new infection rates originating from ONE infected person with OMICRON, DELTA, or the ORIGINAL VERSION of Corona.

CORONA TABLE									CONDENSED version
THEORETICAL WEEKLY NEW COVID-19 INFECTIONS ORIGINATING FROM ONE INFECTED PERSON									
ORIGINAL version	Generation time, days ·		**7.0**		Generation speed (G), Gen/ week -->				**1.00**
Reproduction number (R) >	**1.00**	**1.20**	**1.50**	**1.80**	**2.00**	**2.40**	**3.00**	**3.60**	**4.00**	**4.50**
Week-1	1.0	1.2	1.5	1.8	2.0	2.4	3.0	3.6	4.0	4.5
Week-2	1.0	1.4	2.3	3.2	4.0	6	9	13	16	20
Week-3	1.0	1.7	3.4	5.8	8.0	14	27	47	64	91
Week-4	1.0	2.1	5.1	10.5	16.0	33	81	168	256	410
Last week of Month-1	1.0	2.2	5.8	13	20	44	117	257	406	677
Last week of Month-2	1.0	4.9	34	163	406	1,973	13,647	66,266	165,140	458,327
Last week of Month-3	1.0	10.7	195	2,082	8,192	87,649	1,594,323	17,058,173	67,108,864	310,286,356
Week-to-week growth factor	1.00	1.20	1.50	1.80	2.00	2.40	3.00	3.60	4.00	4.50
Month-to-month growth factor	1.00	2.2	5.8	12.8	20	44	117	257	406	677
Day-to-day growth, %	0.0%	2.6%	6.0%	8.8%	10.4%	13.3%	17.0%	20.1%	21.9%	24.0%
Doubling time, days	Infinity	26.6	12.0	8.3	7.0	5.5	4.4	3.8	3.5	3.2
Doubling time, hours	Infinity	639	287	198	168	133	106	91	84	77
DELTA variant	Generation time, days ·		**5.0**		Generation speed (G), Gen/ week -->				**1.40**
Reproduction number (R) >	**1.00**	**1.20**	**1.50**	**1.80**	**2.00**	**2.40**	**3.00**	**3.60**	**4.00**	**4.50**
Week-1	1.4	1.7	2.3	2.9	3.3	4.1	5.5	6.9	8.0	9.3
Week-2	1.4	2.3	4.0	6.5	8.7	14	26	42	55	76
Week-3	1.4	2.9	7.1	15	23	48	119	250	386	626
Week-4	1.4	3.8	12.6	34	60	163	553	1,505	2,686	5,137
Last week of Month-1	1.4	4.1	15	45	83	245	924	2,736	5,130	10,365
Last week of Month-2	1.4	12.3	178	1,579	5,580	49,703	724,676	6,487,628	23,047,106	95,148,764
Last week of Month-3	1.4	37.3	2,083	55,845	374,039	10,069,317	568,433,270	15,381,112,408	103,541,316,015	873,425,229,886
Week-to-week growth factor	1.00	1.29	1.76	2.28	2.64	3.41	4.66	6.01	6.96	8.21
Month-to-month growth factor	1.00	3.0	11.7	35	67	203	784	2,371	4,493	9,180
Day-to-day growth, %	0.0%	3.7%	8.4%	12.5%	14.9%	19.1%	24.6%	29.2%	32.0%	35.1%
Doubling time, days	Infinity	19.0	8.5	5.9	5.0	4.0	3.2	2.7	2.5	2.3
Doubling time, hours	Infinity	456	205	142	120	95	76	65	60	55
OMICRON variant	Generation time, days ·		**3.5**		Generation speed (G), Gen/ week -->				**2.00**
Reproduction number (R) >	**1.00**	**1.20**	**1.50**	**1.80**	**2.00**	**2.40**	**3.00**	**3.60**	**4.00**	**4.50**
Week-1	2.0	2.6	3.8	5.0	6.0	8.2	12.0	16.6	20.0	24.8
Week-2	2.0	3.8	8.4	16	24	47	108	215	320	501
Week-3	2.0	5.5	19	53	96	271	972	2,781	5,120	10,149
Week-4	2.0	7.9	43	171	384	1,559	8,748	36,048	81,920	205,518
Last week of Month-1	2.0	9	56	254	610	2,795	18,197	84,673	206,425	560,177
Last week of Month-2	2.0	43	1,880	41,363	247,711	5,515,639	248,336,459	5,610,893,312	34,089,178,019	256,744,065,848
Last week of Month-3	2.0	210	63,128	6,744,825	100,663,296	10,883,283,939	3,389,154,437,772	371,809,387,633,792	5,629,499,534,213,120	117,672,649,988,687,000
Week-to-week growth factor	1.00	1.44	2.25	3.24	4.0	5.8	9.0	13.0	16.0	20.3
Month-to-month growth factor	1.00	4.86	34	163	406	1,973	13,647	66,266	165,140	458,327
Day-to-day growth, %	0.0%	5.3%	12.3%	18.3%	21.9%	28.4%	36.9%	44.2%	48.6%	53.7%
Doubling time, days	Infinity	13.3	6.0	4.1	3.5	2.8	2.2	1.9	1.8	1.6
Doubling time, hours	Infinity	319	144	99	84	67	53	45	42	39

Table 4: CONDENSED version, Corona Table: Theoretical WEEKLY new infection rates originating from ONE infected person with OMICRON, DELTA, or the ORIGINAL VERSION of Corona.

CORONA TABLE									JUMP version
THEORETICAL WEEKLY NEW COVID-19 INFECTIONS ORIGINATING FROM ONE INFECTED PERSON									
ORIGINAL version	Generation time, days -		7.0		Generation speed (G), Gen/ week -->				1.00
Reproduction number (R) >	1.00	1.20	1.50	1.80	2.00	2.40	3.00	3.60	4.00	4.50
Week-1	1.0	1.2	1.5	1.8	2.0	2.4	3.0	3.6	4.0	4.5
Week-2	1.0	1.4	2.3	3.2	4.0	6	9	13	16	20
Week-3	1.0	1.7	3.4	5.8	8.0	14	27	47	64	91
Week-4	1.0	2.1	5.1	10.5	16.0	33	81	168	256	410
Last week of Month-1	1.0	2.2	5.8	13	20	44	117	257	406	677
Last week of Month-2	1.0	4.9	34	163	406	1,973	13,647	66,266	165,140	458,327
Last week of Month-3	1.0	10.7	195	2,082	8,192	87,649	1,594,323	17,058,173	67,108,864	310,286,356
Week-to-week growth factor	1.00	1.20	1.50	1.80	2.00	2.40	3.00	3.60	4.00	4.50
Month-to-month growth factor	1.00	2.2	5.8	12.8	20	44	117	257	406	677
Day-to-day growth, %	0.0%	2.6%	6.0%	8.8%	10.4%	13.3%	17.0%	20.1%	21.9%	24.0%
Doubling time, days	Infinity	26.6	12.0	8.3	7.0	5.5	4.4	3.8	3.5	3.2
Doubling time, hours	Infinity	639	287	198	168	133	106	91	84	77
DELTA variant	Generation time, days -		5.0		Generation speed (G), Gen/ week -->				1.40
Reproduction number (R) >	1.00	1.20	1.50	1.80	2.00	2.40	3.00	3.60	4.00	4.50
Week-1	1.4	1.7	2.3	2.9	3.3	4.1	5.5	6.9	8.0	9.3
Week-2	1.4	2.3	4.0	6.5	8.7	14	26	42	55	76
Week-3	1.4	2.9	7.1	15	23	48	119	250	386	626
Week-4	1.4	3.8	12.6	34	60	163	553	1,505	2,686	5,137
Last week of Month-1	1.4	4.1	15	45	83	245	924	2,736	5,130	10,365
Last week of Month-2	1.4	12.3	178	1,579	5,580	49,703	724,676	6,487,628	23,047,106	95,148,764
Last week of Month-3	1.4	37.3	2,083	55,845	374,039	10,069,317	568,433,270	15,381,112,408	103,541,316,015	873,425,229,886
Week-to-week growth factor	1.00	1.29	1.76	2.28	2.64	3.41	4.66	6.01	6.96	8.21
Month-to-month growth factor	1.00	3.0	11.7	35	67	203	784	2,371	4,493	9,180
Day-to-day growth, %	0.0%	3.7%	8.4%	12.5%	14.9%	19.1%	24.6%	29.2%	32.0%	35.1%
Doubling time, days	Infinity	19.0	8.5	5.9	5.0	4.0	3.2	2.7	2.5	2.3
Doubling time, hours	Infinity	456	205	142	120	95	76	65	60	55
OMICRON variant	Generation time, days -		3.5		Generation speed (G), Gen/ week -->				2.00
Reproduction number (R) >	1.00	1.20	1.50	1.80	2.00	2.40	3.00	3.60	4.00	4.50
Week-1	2.0	2.6	3.8	5.0	6.0	8.2	12.0	16.6	20.0	24.8
Week-2	2.0	3.8	8.4	16	24	47	108	215	320	501
Week-3	2.0	5.5	19	53	96	271	972	2,781	5,120	10,149
Week-4	2.0	7.9	43	171	384	1,559	8,748	36,048	81,920	205,518
Last week of Month-1	2.0	9	56	254	610	2,795	18,197	84,673	206,425	560,177
Last week of Month-2	2.0	43	1,880	41,363	247,711	5,515,639	248,336,459	5,610,893,312	34,089,178,019	256,744,065,848
Last week of Month-3	2.0	210	63,128	6,744,825	100,663,296	10,883,283,939	3,389,154,437,772	371,809,387,633,792	5,629,499,534,213,120	117,872,649,988,687,000
Week-to-week growth factor	1.00	1.44	2.25	3.24	4.0	5.8	9.0	13.0	16.0	20.3
Month-to-month growth factor	1.00	4.86	34	163	406	1,973	13,647	66,266	165,140	458,327
Day-to-day growth, %	0.0%	5.3%	12.3%	18.3%	21.9%	28.4%	36.9%	44.2%	48.6%	53.7%
Doubling time, days	Infinity	13.3	6.0	4.1	3.5	2.8	2.2	1.9	1.8	1.6
Doubling time, hours	Infinity	319	144	99	84	67	53	45	42	39

Table 5: JUMP version, Corona Table: Theoretical WEEKLY new infection rates originating from ONE infected person with OMICRON, DELTA, or the ORIGINAL VERSION of Corona. Vertical color codes correspond to the jump from one variant to another.

CORONA TABLE						FUTURE version
THEORETICAL WEEKLY NEW COVID-19 INFECTIONS ORIGINATING FROM ONE INFECTED PERSON						
DELTA variant	Generation time, days -->	5.0		Generation speed (G), Gen/ week -->		1.40
Reproduction number (R) >	1.00	1.20	1.50	2.00	3.00	4.00	4.50

DELTA variant	1.00	1.20	1.50	2.00	3.00	4.00	4.50
Week-1	1.4	1.7	2.3	3.3	5.5	8.0	9.3
Week-2	1.4	2.3	4.0	8.7	26	55	76
Week-3	1.4	2.9	7.1	23	119	386	626
Week-4	1.4	3.8	12.6	60	553	2,686	5,137
Last week of Month-1	1.4	4.1	15	83	924	5,130	10,365
Last week of Month-2	1.4	12.3	178	5,580	724,676	23,047,106	95,148,764
Last week of Month-3	1.4	37.3	2,083	374,039	568,433,270	103,541,316,015	873,425,229,886
Week-to-week growth factor	1.00	1.29	1.76	2.64	4.66	6.96	8.21
Month-to-month growth factor	1.00	3.0	11.7	67	784	4,493	9,180
Day-to-day growth, %	0.0%	3.7%	8.4%	14.9%	24.6%	32.0%	35.1%
Doubling time, days	Infinity	19.0	8.5	5.0	3.2	2.5	2.3
Doubling time, hours	Infinity	456	205	120	76	60	55

OMICRON variant	Generation time, days -->	3.5		Generation speed (G), Gen/ week -->		2.00
Reproduction number (R) >	1.00	1.20	1.50	2.00	3.00	4.00	4.50
Week-1	2.0	2.6	3.8	6.0	12.0	20.0	24.8
Week-2	2.0	3.8	8.4	24	108	320	501
Week-3	2.0	5.5	19	96	972	5,120	10,149
Week-4	2.0	7.9	43	384	8,748	81,920	205,518
Last week of Month-1	2.0	9	56	610	18,197	206,425	560,177
Last week of Month-2	2.0	43	1,880	247,711	248,336,459	34,089,178,019	256,744,065,848
Last week of Month-3	2.0	210	63,128	100,663,296	3,389,154,437,772	5,629,499,534,213,120	117,672,649,988,687,000
Week-to-week growth factor	1.00	1.44	2.25	4.00	9.00	16.00	20.25
Month-to-month growth factor	1.00	4.9	34	406	13,647	165,140	458,327
Day-to-day growth, %	0.0%	5.3%	12.3%	21.9%	36.9%	48.6%	53.7%
Doubling time, days	Infinity	13.3	6.0	3.5	2.2	1.8	1.6
Doubling time, hours	Infinity	319	144	84	53	42	39

FUTURE variant ??	Generation time, days -->	2.5		Generation speed (G), Gen/ week -->		2.80
Reproduction number (R) >	1.00	1.20	1.50	2.00	3.00	4.00	4.50
Week-1	2.8	4.0	6.3	11.9	31.0	63.3	85.4
Week-2	2.8	6.7	20	83	672	3,072	5,763
Week-3	2.8	11.1	61	579	14,568	149,003	388,725
Week-4	2.8	18.5	191	4,029	315,744	7,227,083	26,220,312
Last week of Month-1	2.8	22	279	7,695	880,335	26,356,378	106,734,019
Last week of Month-2	2.8	200	38,188	34,570,659	541,650,528,596	531,961,599,110,808	8,993,899,531,790,660
Last week of Month-3	2.8	1,829	5,230,039	155,311,974,022	333,265,529,070,202,000	10,736,799,529,234,200,000,000	757,867,352,751,923,000,000,000
Week-to-week growth factor	1.00	1.67	3.11	7.0	21.7	48.5	67.5
Month-to-month growth factor	1.00	9.1	137	4,493	615,278	20,183,411	84,264,601
Day-to-day growth, %	0.0%	7.6%	17.6%	32.0%	55.2%	74.1%	82.5%
Doubling time, days	Infinity	9.5	4.3	2.5	1.6	1.3	1.2
Doubling time, hours	Infinity	228	103	60	38	30	28

Table 6: FUTURE version, Corona Table: Theoretical WEEKLY new infection rates originating from ONE infected person with OMICRON, DELTA, and HYPOTHETICAL Future speedier variant with Generation time of 2.5 days/ week.

10.4   A DEMO IN USING THE JUMP VERSION OF CORONA TABLE

Go to Table 5 for the Jump version.

The Reproduction numbers that the table covers are: 1.0, 1.2, 1.5, 1.8, 2.0, 2.4, 3.0, 3.6, 4.0, & 4.5.

Vertical color codes in the table indicate a jump from one variant to another, including the jump to the corresponding Reproduction number and Generation time.

A Demo in reading and interpreting the Corona Table is given below, assuming that the Delta or Omicron variant jumps in to substitute the current variant.

10.4.1   If the Original version is currently dominant

We assume that one person gets infected with the original version of the virus. Therefore, we start with the top section of the Corona Table that covers the original version. Take, for example, the **red column** for Reproduction number **1.50.**

It shows that one infected person will produce 1.5 new infections in the first week, which will lead to 5.1 new infections in the fourth week, 34 new infections in the last week of the second month, and so on.

The week-to-week increase will be 1.5x times and the month-to-month increase 5.8x times. The day-to-day growth will be 6.0%, and the doubling time of new infections will be 12.0 days or 287 hours. These values will also remain constant as long as the other variables such as social behavior and immunization levels also remain unchanged.

10.4.2   If Delta sweeps in

If Delta crashes in and displaces the original version, we need to go to the second block of the table titled Delta and go to the **red column** with Reproduction number **3.0**. The relevant Reproduction number is 3.0 because it doubles when the switch is from the original version to Delta.

In this column, you can see that if one person gets infected with Delta, he will infect 5.5 others in the first week, which will lead to 26 new infections in the second week, 119 new infections in the third week, and so on.

The week-to-week increase will be 4.66x times and the month-to-month increase 784x times. With a daily growth of 24.6%, the doubling time will be only 3.2 days or 76 hours.

If nothing changes, this one single infection will lead to 568 million weekly new infections in the last week of the third month.

10.4.3   If Omicron sweeps in

If Omicron crashes in and displaces Delta, we go to the third and last block of the table titled Omicron and go to the **red column** with Reproduction number **4.5**. The relevant Reproduction number is 4.5 because it increases by 50% (factor 1.5) when the switch is from Delta to Omicron.

In this column, you can see that if one person gets Omicron, he will infect 24.8 others in the first week, which will lead to 501 new infections in the second week, 560,177 new infections in the last week of the first month, and so on.

The week-to-week increase will be 20.3x times and the month-to-month increase 458,327x times. With a daily growth of 53.7%, the doubling time will be only 1.6 days or 39 hours.

If nothing stands in the way, this one single infection will lead to more than half a million weekly new infections in the last week of the first month. But it is unlikely to get that far because additional preventive measures, over and above those already in place to curb the Delta variant, will kick down the Reproduction number from the sky-rocketed 4.5 to a much lower number.

* * * *

11 CORONA FORMULAS: FORMULAS FOR THE GROWTH FACTOR OF WEEKLY INFECTIONS

11.1 THE FORMULAS

> **The formula for the GROWTH FACTOR of WEEKLY new infections = R^G.**

This formula gives the week-on-week growth factor of infections.

In this equation, **R** is the **Reproduction number**, and **G** is the **Generation speed** as defined in section 2 above.

The equation means if we knew the number of new infections last week, the number of new infections this week would be higher by a factor R^G. With respect to the number of infections this week, new infections in the next week will again be higher by a factor R^G. That leads us to another formula as below.

> **The formula for the GROWTH FACTOR of WEEKLY new infections in WEEK N = R^{GN}.**

The above formula is mathematically the same as $(R^G)^N$.

This formula gives the growth factor of weekly infections in week number N.

In the above formulas, G= **1.00** for the **original** version of the virus, G= **1.40** for **Delta**, and G= **2.00** for **Omicron. N** is the number of weeks from your reference point for which you want to know the number of new infections.

The value of R, which represents the average number of people infected by one infector, is estimated and published by the local health authorities based on the actual number of infections.

11.2   EXAMPLES

Example-1: For Omicron, G = 2.0. If Reproduction number R is 3.0, the value of $R^G = 3^2 = 3\times3 = 9.0$. The factor for the week-to-week growth of infections will therefore be 9.0.

Example-2: Assume there are 1,000 Omicron infections in a city this week, and the average Reproduction number is 4.0 because social restrictions were just relaxed by the mayor last week. How many new infections can the mayor expect next week, and how many after 4 weeks?

Applying the first formula, the **growth factor** for next week will be $4^2 = 4\times4 =$ **16**.

Therefore, **new infections** next week will be 16x1,000 =**16,000.**

Applying the second formula, the **growth factor** for the fourth week will be $4^{2\times4} = 4^8 =$ **65,536.**

Therefore, **new infections** in the fourth week will be 65,536 x 1,000 = **65.536 million**!!

If the Generation speed was just 1.0 as was with the original version of the virus, the factor for the week-to-week growth of infections would have been only 4.0 (= 4^1) instead of 16.0, and new infections next week would have been only 4,000 instead of 16,000.

If the Generation speed was just 1.0 instead of 2.0, the growth factor for the 4th week would have been $4^4 = 256$ instead of 65,536, and new infections would have been 0.256 million instead of 65.536 million, a 256-fold difference (= 65,536/ 256).

11.3   THE CORONA BRAKE: WHERE IS THE BRAKE PEDAL?

As the Corona Formulas above show, the Reproduction number R and Generation speed G work together in tandem to determine the weekly growth factor of infections. However, unlike Reproduction number R, the Generation speed **G is variant-specific**, and we humans have **no direct control** over its **value**. It is determined mainly by the mutations of the virus itself. With a speed of 2.0 generations per week, Omicron has a 43% higher speed than Delta and a 100% higher speed than the original version. With 1.40 Generations per week, Delta has a 40% higher speed than the original version.

As is evident from the above examples, the Generation speed G, riding literally on the back of Reproduction number R, can create a disaster if you let R go on a brake-free ride in the community.

> As G is an exponent of R, i.e., as G is riding on the back of R, the impact of G on infection rates depends primarily on the value of R and only secondarily on its own value. The higher the value of R, the higher the impact of G on infection rates and vice versa. If R is small, 1.05, for example, a G with a value of 2.0 (Omicron!) cannot do much havoc, contrary to when R has a value of 4.0 as in the above example.

> But we do have control over the IMPACT of Generation speed G, and that is INDIRECTLY through controlling the value of Reproduction number R. When we bring down the value of R through immunizations and social restrictions, we literally shoot down also the impact of G on infection rates. If R reduces to 1.0 or lower, G becomes as powerless as a powerful rocket without fuel, unable to fly.

> Therefore, the brake pedal, the only one we have, is the R-value. It is a two-in-one pedal though only "R" is marked on it. When infection rates fly beyond control, instead of throwing up our hands in helplessness and blaming G for the havoc, we need to apply the brake of Reproduction number by limiting social contacts and increasing immunization levels if possible.

11.3.1   For Omicron, Reproduction number R is a hyper-brake

As you can see in detail in section 12.3 below, Omicron's infection rate is a lot more sensitive to any change in the value of R compared to Delta. That is because of two reasons.

1. Because the Growth Factor formula is R^G, Omicrons' higher Generation speed G of **2.0** has considerably higher leverage on the infection rate than Delta with its G value of **1.40**. For the original version of the virus, the G value is **1.0**; therefore, it has no leverage.

2. As you can see in detail in section 12.3.2 below, Omicron has a Flipping value of **2.0** against Delta's **5.70**. That means, in the formula R^G for the weekly growth factor of infections, the Generation speed G dominates the infection rate if the value of R is above 2.0, while this lower limit for Delta is 5.70.

The result is that if Omicron is prevailing, any minor change in the Reproduction number R will have a much more amplified effect on the growth rate of infections than is the case with Delta. The impact of R gets amplified irrespective of whether R is moving up or moving down!

> **In practice, it means that if Omicron is prevailing, any relaxation in social behavior will result in a considerably amplified increase in infections. Similarly, any tightening of social behavior will produce amplified results, fooling policymakers to relax too much too quickly after that. However, this amplifying effect will be much less with Delta and totally absent in the case of the original version of the virus.**

With this effect in mind, it is with a bit of concern that I am watching the almost total lifting of social restrictions in some European countries, especially the UK. It is like taking the foot off the brake with a steep slope and a ravine downhill. But, of course, the emergency handbrake is there to save the bus!

* * * *

12 THE RELATIVE SHARES OF REPRODUCTION NUMBER R AND GENERATION SPEED G ON INFECTION RATES

12.1 REPRODUCTION NUMBER R

The notation for Reproduction number is **R.**

Based on all the data available in the public domain, we have assumed the following.

If **Delta** displaces the original version, the Reproduction number R will **double** in value if immunization levels and social behavior remain unchanged.

If **Omicron** displaces the original version, the Reproduction number R will **triple** in value if immunization levels and social behavior remain unchanged.

It follows automatically from the above that, if **Omicron displaces Delta**, the Reproduction number R will increase by **50%** (factor 1.5) if nothing else changes.

12.2 GENERATION SPEED G

The original version of the virus had a Generation time of **7 days** or one transmission cycle per week. That means it took an average of 7 days for one infected person to infect another person.

The Generation **time** decreased to **5 days for Delta** and **3.5 days for Omicron**. That means there will be 1.4 Generations per week for Delta and 2.0 Generations per week for Omicron.

The Generation **speed** G for the original version is **1.0** generation per week, G for Delta is **1.4** generations per week, and G for Omicron is **2.0** generations per week.

12.3   WHAT CAUSES MORE INFECTIONS: THE HIGH REPRODUCTION NUMBER OR THE HIGH GENERATION SPEEDS OF DELTA AND OMICRON?

It is helpful to know which of the two factors is causing comparatively more infections so that containment measures can be adapted accordingly. We can use the Corona Tables to check it or calculate it precisely using the Growth Code.

12.3.1   Comparing the comparative share of infections using the Corona Table

12.3.1.1   The share of Reproduction number R on infection rates

It can be seen at a glance in the Corona Table by following and comparing values in any **horizontal row** in the **same block**. All horizontal rows in the same block, going from left to right, have the same value of Generation speed, leaving R as the only variable. Therefore, by going from left to right in the same row, the values can be easily compared for the impact of R.

Example: Let us go to Table 4 and the row for week 4. The growth factor for Reproduction number 1.5 is **5.1**. Moving to the right in the same row, we get **81** as the growth factor if R is 3.0. Moving further to the right in the same row, we get **410** as the growth factor if R is 4.5. These increases are purely due to the rise in the Reproduction number with nothing else changed.

12.3.1.2   The share of Generation speed G on infection rates

It can be seen at a glance in the Corona Table by following any **vertical column** and comparing corresponding values in the **different blocks.** All vertical columns have the same R-value, leaving G as the only variable between the three blocks. Therefore, the corresponding values in each row can be compared for the impact of G.

Example: Let us go to Table 4 again and to the column for R 1.5 and the growth factors for week 4. The growth factor for Reproduction number 1.5 is **5.1** for the original version of the virus. Moving down in the same column to week 4 in the Delta block, we get **12.6** as the growth factor. Moving further down to week 4 for Omicron, we get **43.0** as the growth factor. These increases are purely due to the increase of Generation speed with nothing else changed.

Please note that this example and comparison are purely for the purpose of illustrating the impact of G on growth factors. In reality, the corresponding column for Delta would be for R 3.0 because of the doubling of R, and for Omicron, it would be the column for R 4.5 because of the tripling of R.

12.3.2   Comparing the relative share of infections by calculation

In section 11 above, we have seen that the weekly growth rate of infections is determined by the formula R^G.

12.3.2.1   Omicron and its Flipping value

If we analyze the weekly growth factor of infections for Omicron, which is given by the formula R^G, we get the following.

> **2.0 is the Flipping value for R. That means if R is 2.0 for Omicron, Reproduction number and Generation speed contribute equally to the growth of infections.**

That follows from the following calculation.

$R^G = 2^2 = 2 \times 2 = 4.0$

Of the 4-fold weekly increase of infections, 2-fold increase is due to R's value, and 2-fold increase is due to G's value.

If the value of **R is lower than 2.0**, the share of R in the growth of infections will be more than that of G.

For example, if R has a value of 1.5, the factor for the total increase of weekly infections = R^G =1.5^2 = 1.5 x 1.5 = 2.25.

Of this, factor 1.5 is caused by R, and the remaining 0.75 is caused by G.

> **The lower the value of R, paradoxically, the higher the share of R in the weekly infections and the lower the share of G.**

If the value of **R is higher than the flipping value of 2.0**, the share of G in the growth of infections will be more than that of R.

For example, if R has a value of 3.0, the factor for the total increase of weekly infections = R^G = 3^2 = 3 x 3 = 9.

Of this, factor 3.0 is caused by R, and the remaining 6.0 is caused by G, 2-fold higher than that of R.

Similarly, if R has a value of 4.0, the factor for the total increase of weekly infections will be 16.0, of which the share of R will be 4.0, and the share of G will be 12.0. The share of G is 3-fold higher than that of R.

Similarly, if R has a value of 5.0, the factor for the total increase of weekly infections will be 25.0, of which the share of R will be 5.0, and the share of G will be 20.0. The share of G is 4-fold higher than that of R.

> **The higher the value of R, paradoxically, the lower the share of R in the weekly infections and the higher the share of G.**

12.3.2.2   Delta and its Flipping value

If we analyze the weekly growth factor of infections for Delta, which is given by the formula R^G, we get the following.

> **5.7 is the Flipping value for R. That means if R is 5.7 for Delta, Reproduction number and Generation speed contribute equally to the growth of infections.**

That follows from the following calculation.

$R^G = 5.7^{1.4} = 11.40$

Of the 11.4-fold weekly increase of infections, 5.7-fold increase is due to R's value, and 5.7-fold increase is due to G's value.

If the value of **R is lower than 5.7**, the share of R in the growth of infections will be more than that of G.

For example, if R has a value of 4.0, the factor for the total increase of weekly infections = $R^G = 4^{1.4} = 7.0$.

Of this, factor 4.0 is caused by R, and the remaining 3.0 is caused by G.

> As is the case also with Omicron, the lower the value of R, paradoxically, the higher the share of R in the weekly infections and the lower the share of G.

If the value of **R is higher than the flipping value of 5.7**, the share of G will be more than that of R.

For example, if R has a value of 7.0, the factor for the total increase of weekly infections = $R^G = 7^{1.4} = 15.20$.

Of this, the factor 7.0 is caused by R, and the remaining 8.2 is caused by G.

Similarly, if R has a value of 8.0, the factor for the total increase of weekly infections will be 18.4, of which the share of R will be 8.0, and the share of G will be 10.40.

Similarly, if R has a value of 9.0, the factor for the total increase of weekly infections will be 21.7, of which the share of R will be 9.0, and the share of G will be 12.70.

> As is the case also with Omicron, the higher the value of R, paradoxically, the lower the share of R in the weekly infections and the higher the share of G.

12.4   CONCLUSIONS

From the above, it is clear that, for both Omicron and Delta, there is a flipping point in the value of Reproduction number R at which the share of Reproduction number R and share of Generation speed G in the total number of weekly infections are equal.

The flipping point for the value of R for **Omicron** is **2.0**.

The flipping point for the value of R for **Delta** is **5.7.**

If the value of R is above the flipping point, paradoxically, G becomes more dominant, and the share of G becomes more than that of R.

If the value of R is below the flipping point, paradoxically, R itself becomes more dominant, and the share of G becomes less than that of R.

The paradox that the higher the value of R, the lower its own share and the higher the share of G in the total number of weekly infections applies at all times and to both Omicron and Delta.

* * * *

13 REASONS WHY OMICRON SPREADS MUCH FASTER THAN DELTA

From a mathematical perspective, the reasons can be summed up as below based on what we have analyzed and the conclusions drawn from the chapters above.

13.1 THE REASONS FOR OMICRON'S MUCH FASTER GROWTH RATE

> **With Omicron, the Reproduction number R makes a 3-fold leap compared to the original version, while Delta's leap is only 2-fold.**

> **Omicron has the highest Generation speed G of 2.0 generations per week compared to 1.4 for Delta and 1.0 for the original version.**

In other words, the Generation period for Omicron is 3.5 days, for Delta it is 5.0 days, and for the original version it is 7.0 days.

> **As you can see also in the examples below, this increased Generation speed is the main cause of the explosive growth of Omicron whenever the Reproduction number shoots above 2.0.**

> **If the Reproduction number is under 2.0, the Reproduction number itself becomes the leading contributor to infections, and the growth rate will be relatively modest.**

The growth factor for weekly infections is given by the formula R^G. The flipping point for the value of R, at which point G becomes more dominant than R, lies at 2.0 for Omicron, much lower than the 5.7 for Delta.

While Omicron's G with a turbo-power of 2.0 takes the driver's seat as early as 2.0 for the value of R, Delta's G with a smaller turbo-power of only 1.4 takes the driver's seat as late as 5.7 for the value of R. Therefore, the speeds become incomparable. Let us take three examples to demonstrate the above statements.

13.2　EXAMPLE 13.2:　THE ORIGINAL VERSION PREVAILS BEFORE OMICRON CRASHES IN

Let us assume the prevailing value of R was **1.5** before Omicron or Delta displaced it. The Generation speed for the original version is **1.0** generation per week.

The growth rate of weekly infections with the **original version** = R^G = 1.5^1 = **1.50x**

Omicron displaces the original version

When Omicron arrives, the value of R jumps 3-fold from 1.5 to 4.5.

The Generation speed increases from 1.0 generation per week to 2.0 generations.

The new growth rate of weekly infections with **Omicron** = R^G = 4.5^2 = **20.25x**

With the arrival of Omicron in a community with the original version of the virus, the weekly growth rate of infections exploded from **1.5**-fold per week to **20.25**-fold per week.

In a city with 1,000 new infections with the original version last week, and you were anticipating it would increase to 1,500 this week because the Reproduction number was 1.50, you will get to deal with 20,250 new infections this week due to Omicron. This is **13.5-fold** (= 20.25/ 1.5) **more infections in a week than was anticipated** with the original version, and it is caused by Omicron. The **Jump factor, in this case,** is **13.5x**

Of this **20.25**-fold growth in a week compared to the previous week, only **4.5**-fold is caused by **R**, and the remaining **15.75**-fold is caused by **G**. That means the share of G in the weekly infections is **77.8%,** and that of R is **22.2%**.

The main culprit for the explosive growth of infections in this example is, therefore, the shortened Generation time (or the increased Generation speed) of Omicron (77.8% share), and the share of Reproduction number R is relatively small (22.2% share).

13.3 EXAMPLE 13.3: THE ORIGINAL VERSION PREVAILS BEFORE DELTA CRASHES IN

As in example 13.2 above, let us assume the prevailing value of R was **1.5** before Omicron or Delta displaced it. The Generation speed for the original version is **1.0** generation per week.

The growth rate of weekly infections with the **original version** = R^G = 1.5^1 = **1.50x**

Delta displaces the original version

When Delta arrives, the value of R jumps 2-fold from 1.5 to 3.0.

The Generation speed increases from 1.0 generation per week to 1.4 generations.

The new growth rate of weekly infections with **Delta** = R^G = $3.0^{1.4}$ = **4.66x**

With the arrival of Delta in a community with the original version of the virus, the weekly growth rate of infections increased from **1.5**-fold per week to **4.66**-fold per week.

In a city with 1,000 new infections with the original version last week, and you anticipated it would increase to 1,500 this week, you will have to deal with 4,660 new infections this week due to Delta. This is **3.1-fold** (= 4.66/ 1.5) **more infections in a week than was anticipated** with the original version, and it is caused by Delta. The **Jump factor, in this case, is 3.1x**

Of this **4.66**-fold growth in a week compared to the previous week, **3.0**-fold is caused by **R**, and only the remaining **1.66**-fold is caused by **G**. That means the share of G in the weekly infections is only **36.0%,** and that of R is **64.0%.**

The main culprit for the growth of infections in this example is the Reproduction number R (64% share), and the share of the increased Generation speed of Delta is relatively small (36% share).

13.4   EXAMPLE 13.4:   DELTA PREVAILS BEFORE OMICRON CRASHES IN

Let us assume that Delta was the prevalent variant, and the prevailing value of R was **3.0** before Omicron came to displace it. The Generation speed for Delta is **1.4** generations per week.

The prevailing growth rate of weekly infections with **Delta** = R^G = $3.0^{1.4}$ = **4.66x**

This situation is also the final situation we had reached in example 13.3 **above**. So now we will let Omicron come in and displace Delta.

Omicron displaces Delta

When Omicron arrives, the value of R jumps 1.5-fold from 3.0 to 4.5.

The Generation speed increases from 1.4 generations per week to 2.0 generations per week.

The new growth rate of weekly infections with **Omicron** = R^G = 4.5^2 = **20.25x.**

This situation is also the final situation we had reached in example 13.2 **above.**

With the arrival of Omicron in a community with Delta, the weekly growth rate of infections increased from **4.66**-fold per week to **20.25**-fold per week.

In a city with 1,000 new infections with Delta last week, and you anticipated it would increase to 4,660 this week, you will get to deal with 20,250 new infections this week due to Omicron. This is **4.3-fold** (= 20.25/ 4.66) **more infections in a week than was anticipated** with Delta, and it is all caused by Omicron. The **Jump factor**, **in this case**, is **4.3x.**

Of this **20.25**-fold growth in a week compared to the previous week, **4.5**-fold is caused by **R**, and **G** causes the remaining 15.75-fold. That means, as was also the case in example 13.2 above, the share of G in the weekly infections is **77.8%,** and that of R is **22.2%**.

The main culprit for the growth of infections in this example is the increased Generation speed G of Omicron (77.8% share), and the share of Reproduction number R is relatively small (22.2% share).

* * * *

14   INFECTION RATE OF OMICRON OR ANY VARIANT IS NOT DEPENDENT ON WHICH VARIANT IT REPLACES

It does not make any difference for the **actual infection numbers,** whether the jump is directly from the original version to Omicron or from Delta to Omicron. It is only the **difference** in weekly infection rates that will be considerably bigger if the jump to Omicron is directly from the original version instead of from Delta. The difference is bigger because the jump in Reproduction number will be 3.0-fold instead of 1.5-fold, and the jump in Generation speed will be 100% instead of 43%. In either case, the number of weekly infections and other results will be the same if all other parameters like immunization levels and social restrictions are also the same.

Jumping to Omicron directly from the original version or through Delta is akin to jumping to the first floor of a building directly from the third floor or jumping to the second floor first and then to the first floor. Of course, you will land on the first floor in either case, but the jump directly from the third floor will be a much harsher experience.

In section 14.1 below, you can see the mathematical validation of the above statement.

14.1   EXAMPLE 14.1

From example 13.2 above, we can see that when **Omicron** displaced the **original version,** which was prevailing with a Reproduction number of 1.50, the weekly growth rate of infections increased from 1.5 to 20.25, or the **Jump factor** was **13.5** (= 20.25/ 1.5).

From example 13.3 above, we can see that when **Delta** displaced the **original version,** which was prevailing with a reproduction number of 1.50, the weekly growth rate of infections increased from 1.5 to 4.66, or the **Jump factor** was **3.1** (= 4.66/ 1.5).

From example 13.4 above, we can see that when **Omicron** displaced **Delta,** which was prevailing with a reproduction number of 3.0 and Generation speed of 1.4, the weekly growth rate of infections increased from 4.66 to 20.25, or the **Jump factor** was **4.3** (= 20.25/ 4.66). The prevailing Reproduction number of 3.0 and Generation speed of 1.4 with Delta were the direct effect of the transition from the original version to Delta because immunization levels and social restrictions remained unchanged even after Delta had displaced the original version.

For the transition from the original version to Omicron via the intermediate step of Delta, we can "mathematically add up" the individual growth factors of the first step from the original version to Delta and the second step from Delta to Omicron. "Mathematically adding up" in this case is done by multiplying one value with the other. Let us do it.

The **Jump factor** of infection rates in the first step of Delta displacing the original version was **3.1.**

The **Jump factor** of infection rates in the second step of Omicron displacing Delta was **4.3.**

The combined **Jump factor** of infection rates of the above two steps = **3.1 x 4.3 = 13.5**

13.5 is precisely the **Jump factor** of infection rates when Omicron had displaced the original version, as in example 13.2 above.

> **From the above, we can infer that the route that Omicron, or any variant, takes to establish itself in a community does not change its behavior or transmissibility.**

* * * *

15   THREE REASONS WHY OMICRON COMES WITH A SHOCK WAVE IN SOME COUNTRIES AND MAKES A MILD ENTRY IN OTHERS

15.1   REASON 1: IT MAY HAVE COME SPLIT INTO 2 PARTS, FIRST DELTA, THEN OMICRON

As seen in the examples above, if Omicron displaces the original version, the jump in the weekly growth factor is 13.5-fold. But if it replaces Delta, the jump in weekly growth factors is only 4.3. The 13.5-fold jump will be experienced as a shock wave compared to the 4.3-fold jump.

The point to note here is that before Omicron came to displace Delta, the community had already undergone the first jump in infection rates when Delta had replaced the original version. As shown in example 13.2 above, they had then experienced a 3.1-fold jump in weekly growth rates. That was the first step. Now they experience the second step with a 4.3-fold jump in growth rates.

In effect, the shock wave of 13.5-fold jump in weekly growth rates came for them split into two smaller jumps of 3.1 and 4.3 each with a time interval between them. Therefore, they did not experience a 13.5-fold jump in growth rate at once even though the final result was the same: a 13.5-fold jump in the weekly growth rate of infections.

In a way, it is akin to increasing an amount 3-fold first and then increasing it 4-fold. The total increase will be 12-fold but not felt as such, unlike a straight 12-fold increase.

15.2   REASON 2: STRICTER PRE-OMICRON SOCIAL BEHAVIOR AND IMMUNIZATION

As we have seen in section 11 and the growth rate formula R^G, the reproduction number R is the only parameter we can control to reduce the infection rates. By controlling R, we can also control the power of the turbo-powered Generation speed G.

Some communities are better at limiting social contacts than others, and some are negligent with it. Suppose R is already high, for example, 3.0 with the original version of the virus prevailing. In that case, when Omicron arrives and slings it 3-fold up to 9.0 and installs the Generation speed G of 2.0 on top of it, it guarantees a shockwave. The weekly growth rate will jump 9-fold.

Communities that have been able to keep the Reproduction number relatively low even before the arrival of Omicron will be spared of such a magnitude 9 shock.

Those communities already dealing with Delta are likely to have stricter social restrictions already in place and a lower pre-Omicron Reproduction number than those still dealing with the less transmissible original version. Due to the low pre-Omicron Reproduction number, these communities will benefit from a lower growth rate when Omicron strikes.

15.3   REASON 3: FOR OMICRON, ANY CHANGE IN REPRODUCTION NUMBER AMPLIFIES INFECTION RATES SIGNIFICANTLY

As you can see in detail in section 11.3.1 above, Omicron's infection rate is a lot more sensitive to any change in the value of R compared to Delta or the original version of the virus. The consequence is that any increase in the Reproduction number, especially if it had already been relatively high, can considerably amplify the growth factor of infections.

Example:

With the formula R^{GN} for the growth factor in mind, suppose the R-value goes up from **2.0** to **4.0** due to the lifting of social restrictions.

As a consequence, the growth factor for weekly infections will jump from **4.0** (=2^2) to **16.0** (=4^2) in the first week, from **16** (=2^4) to **256** (=4^4) in the second week, and from **64** (=2^6) to **4,096** (=4^6) in the third week.

If the increase in the Reproduction number from 2.0 to 4.0 was for Delta or the original version, the weekly growth of infections would have been much lower, as shown below.

1st week: **16x** more infections for Omicron versus **7x** for Delta versus **4x** for the original version.

2nd week: **256x** for Omicron versus **49x** for Delta versus **16x** for the original version.

3rd week: **4096x** for Omicron versus **338x** for Delta versus **64x** for the original version.

As can be seen above, the jump in week-on-week infections is **16**-fold for Omicron, **7**-fold for Delta, and **4**-fold for the original version, even though the increase in the Reproduction number was the same for all three variants. This difference is due to the difference in the value of Generation speed **G** between the three variants when applied to the formula R^{GN}.

This difference in week-on-week infections rates gets amplified again with every passing week. Omicron had a 4-fold higher jump in infection rates than the original version in the first week, but it grew to a **16**-fold difference in the second week and a **64**-fold difference in the third week. This difference is due to the role of time factor **N** in the formula R^{GN}, which is mathematically the same as $(R^{G})^{N}$.

* * * *

16   APPENDIX- A: CORONA TABLES

CORONA TABLE									Page 1
THEORETICAL WEEKLY NEW COVID-19 INFECTIONS ORIGINATING FROM ONE INFECTED PERSON									
ORIGINAL version — Generation time, days --> 7.0				Generation speed (G), Gen/ week -->					1.00
Reproduction number (R) >	0.70	0.80	0.90	0.95	1.00	1.05	1.10	1.15	1.20	1.25
Week-1	0.70	0.80	0.90	0.95	1.00	1.05	1.10	1.15	1.20	1.25
Week-2	0.49	0.64	0.81	0.90	1.00	1.10	1.21	1.32	1.44	1.56
Week-3	0.34	0.51	0.73	0.86	1.00	1.16	1.33	1.52	1.73	1.95
Week-4	0.24	0.41	0.66	0.81	1.00	1.22	1.46	1.75	2.07	2.44
Last week of Month-1	0.21	0.38	0.63	0.80	1.00	1.24	1.51	1.83	2.20	2.63
Last week of Month-2	0.05	0.14	0.40	0.64	1.00	1.5	2.3	3.4	4.9	6.9
Last week of Month-3	0.01	0.05	0.25	0.51	1.00	1.9	3.5	6.2	10.7	18.2
Week-to-week growth factor	0.70	0.80	0.90	0.95	1.00	1.05	1.10	1.15	1.20	1.25
Month-to-month growth factor	0.21	0.38	0.63	0.80	1.00	1.24	1.51	1.83	2.20	2.63
Day-to-day growth, %	-5.0%	-3.1%	-1.5%	-0.7%	0.0%	0.7%	1.4%	2.0%	2.6%	3.2%
Doubling/ halving time, days	-13.6	-21.7	-46.1	-94.6	Infinity	99.4	50.9	34.7	26.6	21.7
Doubling/ halving time, hours	-326	-522	-1,105	-2,270	Infinity	2,387	1,222	833	639	522
DELTA variant — Generation time, days --> 5.0				Generation speed (G), Gen/ week -->					1.40
Reproduction number (R) >	0.70	0.80	0.90	0.95	1.00	1.05	1.10	1.15	1.20	1.25
Week-1	0.92	1.07	1.23	1.32	1.40	1.48	1.57	1.66	1.74	1.83
Week-2	0.56	0.79	1.07	1.23	1.40	1.59	1.79	2.02	2.25	2.51
Week-3	0.34	0.57	0.92	1.14	1.40	1.70	2.05	2.45	2.91	3.42
Week-4	0.21	0.42	0.79	1.06	1.40	1.82	2.34	2.98	3.75	4.68
Last week of Month-1	0.17	0.38	0.75	1.04	1.40	1.86	2.45	3.18	4.09	5.19
Last week of Month-2	0.02	0.10	0.40	0.76	1.40	2.5	4.4	7.4	12.3	20.1
Last week of Month-3	0.00	0.03	0.21	0.56	1.40	3.4	7.8	17.3	37.3	77.9
Week-to-week growth factor	0.61	0.73	0.86	0.93	1.00	1.07	1.14	1.22	1.29	1.37
Month-to-month growth factor	0.11	0.26	0.53	0.73	1.00	1.34	1.78	2.33	3.02	3.87
Day-to-day growth, %	-6.9%	-4.4%	-2.1%	-1.0%	0.0%	1.0%	1.9%	2.8%	3.7%	4.6%
Doubling/ halving time, days	-9.7	-15.5	-32.9	-67.6	Infinity	71.0	36.4	24.8	19.0	15.5
Doubling/ halving time, hours	-233	-373	-789	-1,622	Infinity	1,705	873	595	456	373
OMICRON variant — Generation time, days --> 3.5				Generation speed (G), Gen/ week -->					2.00
Reproduction number (R) >	0.70	0.80	0.90	0.95	1.00	1.05	1.10	1.15	1.20	1.25
Week-1	1.19	1.44	1.71	1.85	2.00	2.15	2.31	2.47	2.64	2.81
Week-2	0.58	0.92	1.39	1.67	2.00	2.37	2.80	3.27	3.80	4.39
Week-3	0.29	0.59	1.12	1.51	2.00	2.62	3.38	4.32	5.47	6.87
Week-4	0.14	0.38	0.91	1.36	2.00	2.88	4.09	5.72	7.88	10.73
Last week of Month-1	0.11	0.33	0.85	1.32	2.00	2.98	4.36	6.28	8.90	12.45
Last week of Month-2	0.01	0.05	0.34	0.84	2.00	4.5	10	21	43	86
Last week of Month-3	0.00	0.01	0.14	0.54	2.00	6.9	23	71	210	596
Week-to-week growth factor	0.49	0.64	0.81	0.90	1.00	1.10	1.21	1.32	1.44	1.56
Month-to-month growth factor	0.05	0.14	0.40	0.64	1.00	1.53	2.28	3.36	4.86	6.92
Day-to-day growth, %	-9.7%	-6.2%	-3.0%	-1.5%	0.0%	1.4%	2.8%	4.1%	5.3%	6.6%
Doubling/ halving time, days	-6.8	-10.9	-23.0	-47.3	Infinity	49.7	25.5	17.4	13.3	10.9
Doubling/ halving time, hours	-163	-261	-553	-1,135	Infinity	1,193	611	417	319	261

Corona Table, page 1: Theoretical **WEEKLY new infection rates** originating from **ONE** infected person with **OMICRON, DELTA**, or the **ORIGINAL VERSION** of Corona.

CORONA TABLE							Page 2
THEORETICAL WEEKLY NEW COVID-19 INFECTIONS ORIGINATING FROM ONE INFECTED PERSON							
ORIGINAL version — Generation time, days --> 7.0 — Gneration speed (G), Gen/ week --> 1.00							
Reproduction number (R) >	1.30	1.40	1.50	1.60	1.70	1.80	1.90	2.00
Week-1	1.30	1.40	1.50	1.60	1.70	1.80	1.90	2.00
Week-2	1.69	1.96	2.25	2.56	2.89	3.24	3.61	4.00
Week-3	2.20	2.74	3.38	4.10	4.91	5.83	6.86	8.00
Week-4	2.86	3.84	5.06	6.55	8.35	10.50	13.03	16.00
Last week of Month-1	3.1	4.3	5.8	7.7	10	13	16	20
Last week of Month-2	10	18	34	59	99	163	261	406
Last week of Month-3	30	79	195	450	990	2,082	4,205	8,192
Week-to-week growth factor	1.30	1.40	1.50	1.60	1.70	1.80	1.90	2.00
Month-to-month growth factor	3.1	4.3	5.8	7.7	10.0	12.8	16.1	20.2
Day-to-day growth, %	3.8%	4.9%	6.0%	6.9%	7.9%	8.8%	9.6%	10.4%
Doubling time, days	18.5	14.4	12.0	10.3	9.1	8.3	7.6	7.0
Doubling time, hours	444	346	287	248	219	198	181	168

DELTA variant — Generation time, days --> 5.0 — Gneration speed (G), Gen/ week --> 1.40							
Reproduction number (R) >	1.30	1.40	1.50	1.60	1.70	1.80	1.90	2.00
Week-1	1.9	2.1	2.3	2.5	2.7	2.9	3.1	3.3
Week-2	2.8	3.4	4.0	4.8	5.6	6.5	7.6	8.7
Week-3	4.0	5.4	7.1	9	12	15	19	23
Week-4	5.8	8.7	12.6	18	25	34	46	60
Last week of Month-1	6.5	10	15	22	32	45	61	83
Last week of Month-2	32	78	178	385	796	1,579	3,018	5,580
Last week of Month-3	158	600	2,083	6,670	19,910	55,845	148,176	374,039
Week-to-week growth factor	1.44	1.60	1.76	1.93	2.10	2.28	2.46	2.64
Month-to-month growth factor	4.9	7.7	11.7	17.3	25	35	49	67
Day-to-day growth, %	5.4%	7.0%	8.4%	9.9%	11.2%	12.5%	13.7%	14.9%
Doubling time, days	13.2	10.3	8.5	7.4	6.5	5.9	5.4	5.0
Doubling time, hours	317	247	205	177	157	142	130	120

OMICRON variant — Generation time, days --> 3.5 — Gneration speed (G), Gen/ week --> 2.00							
Reproduction number (R) >	1.30	1.40	1.50	1.60	1.70	1.80	1.90	2.00
Week-1	3.0	3.4	3.8	4.2	4.6	5.0	5.5	6.0
Week-2	5.1	6.6	8.4	10.6	13	16	20	24
Week-3	8.5	12.9	19	27	38	53	72	96
Week-4	14.4	25.3	43	70	111	171	259	384
Last week of Month-1	17	32	56	95	158	254	398	610
Last week of Month-2	167	585	1,880	5,610	15,681	41,363	103,603	247,711
Last week of Month-3	1,623	10,800	63,128	329,589	1,558,069	6,744,825	26,992,184	100,663,296
Week-to-week growth factor	1.69	1.96	2.25	2.56	2.89	3.24	3.61	4.00
Month-to-month growth factor	9.7	18.5	33.6	59	99	163	261	406
Day-to-day growth, %	7.8%	10.1%	12.3%	14.4%	16.4%	18.3%	20.1%	21.9%
Doubling time, days	9.2	7.2	6.0	5.2	4.6	4.1	3.8	3.5
Doubling time, hours	222	173	144	124	110	99	91	84

Corona Table page 2: Theoretical WEEKLY new infection rates originating from ONE infected person with OMICRON, DELTA, or the ORIGINAL VERSION of Corona.

CORONA TABLE						Page 3
THEORETICAL WEEKLY NEW COVID-19 INFECTIONS ORIGINATING FROM ONE INFECTED PERSON						
ORIGINAL version	Generation time, days -->		7.0	Generation speed (G), Gen/ week -->		1.00
Reproduction number (R) >	2.10	2.20	2.30	2.40	2.50	2.60	2.70
Week-1	2.10	2.20	2.3	2.4	2.5	2.6	2.7
Week-2	4.41	4.84	5.3	5.8	6.3	6.8	7.3
Week-3	9.26	10.65	12.2	13.8	15.6	17.6	19.7
Week-4	19.45	23.43	28	33	39	46	53
Last week of Month-1	25	30	37	44	53	63	74
Last week of Month-2	620	928	1,365	1,973	2,811	3,949	5,476
Last week of Month-3	15,447	28,281	50,404	87,649	149,012	248,115	405,256
Week-to-week growth factor	2.10	2.20	2.30	2.40	2.50	2.60	2.70
Month-to-month growth factor	24.9	30.5	37	44	53	63	74
Day-to-day growth, %	11.2%	11.9%	12.6%	13.3%	14.0%	14.6%	15.2%
Doubling time, days	6.5	6.2	5.8	5.5	5.3	5.1	4.9
Doubling time, hours	157	148	140	133	127	122	117

DELTA variant	Generation time, days -->		5.0	Generation speed (G), Gen/ week -->		1.40
Reproduction number (R) >	2.10	2.20	2.30	2.40	2.50	2.60	2.70
Week-1	3.5	3.7	3.9	4.1	4.3	4.6	4.8
Week-2	9.8	11.1	12.5	14.1	15.7	17.4	19.2
Week-3	28	34	40	48	57	66	77
Week-4	79	101	129	163	204	253	311
Last week of Month-1	111	146	191	245	313	395	494
Last week of Month-2	10,016	17,499	29,826	49,703	81,128	129,915	204,395
Last week of Month-3	902,632	2,091,095	4,667,447	10,069,317	21,054,272	42,772,345	84,607,974
Week-to-week growth factor	2.83	3.02	3.2	3.4	3.6	3.8	4.0
Month-to-month growth factor	90	119	156	203	260	329	414
Day-to-day growth, %	16.0%	17.1%	18.1%	19.1%	20.1%	21.1%	22.0%
Doubling time, days	4.7	4.4	4.2	4.0	3.8	3.6	3.5
Doubling time, hours	112	105	100	95	91	87	84

OMICRON variant	Generation time, days -->		3.5	Generation speed (G), Gen/ week -->		2.00
Reproduction number (R) >	2.10	2.20	2.30	2.40	2.50	2.60	2.70
Week-1	6.5	7.0	7.6	8.2	8.8	9.4	10.0
Week-2	29	34	40	47	55	63	73
Week-3	127	165	212	271	342	428	531
Week-4	558	798	1,124	1,559	2,136	2,891	3,870
Last week of Month-1	916	1,350	1,958	2,795	3,935	5,467	7,505
Last week of Month-2	567,907	1,253,296	2,671,377	5,515,639	11,059,993	21,587,409	41,096,976
Last week of Month-3	352,244,371	1,163,367,692	3,645,103,299	10,883,283,939	31,086,244,690	85,238,578,803	225,058,711,454
Week-to-week growth factor	4.41	4.84	5.3	5.8	6.3	6.8	7.3
Month-to-month growth factor	620	928	1,365	1,973	2,811	3,949	5,476
Day-to-day growth, %	23.6%	25.3%	26.9%	28.4%	29.9%	31.4%	32.8%
Doubling time, days	3.3	3.1	2.9	2.8	2.6	2.5	2.4
Doubling time, hours	78	74	70	67	64	61	59

Corona Table, page 3: Theoretical WEEKLY new infection rates originating from ONE infected person with OMICRON, DELTA, or the ORIGINAL VERSION of Corona.

CORONA TABLE						Page 4
THEORETICAL WEEKLY NEW COVID-19 INFECTIONS ORIGINATING FROM ONE INFECTED PERSON						
ORIGINAL version	Generation time, days -->	7.0		Generation speed (G), Gen/ week		1.00
Reproduction number (R) >	2.80	2.90	3.00	3.20	3.40	3.50	3.60
Week-1	2.8	2.9	3.0	3.2	3.4	3.5	3.6
Week-2	7.8	8.4	9.0	10.2	11.6	12	13
Week-3	22.0	24.4	27.0	32.8	39.3	43	47
Week-4	61	71	81	105	134	150	168
Last week of Month-1	87	101	117	155	201	228	257
Last week of Month-2	7,505	10,173	13,647	23,876	40,379	51,911	66,266
Last week of Month-3	650,211	1,026,063	1,594,323	3,689,349	8,113,830	11,827,272	17,058,173
Week-to-week growth factor	2.80	2.90	3.00	3.20	3.40	3.50	3.60
Month-to-month growth factor	87	101	117	155	201	228	257
Day-to-day growth, %	15.8%	16.4%	17.0%	18.1%	19.1%	19.6%	20.1%
Doubling time, days	4.7	4.6	4.4	4.2	4.0	3.9	3.8
Doubling time, hours	113	109	106	100	95	93	91
DELTA variant	Generation time, days -->	5.0		Generation speed (G), Gen/ week		1.40
Reproduction number (R) >	2.80	2.90	3.00	3.20	3.40	3.50	3.60
Week-1	5.0	5.3	5.5	6.0	6.4	6.7	6.9
Week-2	21.2	23.3	25.5	30.4	35.7	39	42
Week-3	90	103	119	155	198	223	250
Week-4	379	459	553	788	1,100	1,289	1,505
Last week of Month-1	613	755	924	1,357	1,946	2,313	2,736
Last week of Month-2	316,349	482,216	724,676	1,574,005	3,262,481	4,623,154	6,487,628
Last week of Month-3	163,276,997	307,932,791	568,433,270	1,826,344,424	5,468,314,230	9,238,848,151	15,381,112,408
Week-to-week growth factor	4.2	4.4	4.7	5.1	5.5	5.8	6.0
Month-to-month growth factor	516	639	784	1,160	1,676	1,998	2,371
Day-to-day growth, %	22.9%	23.7%	24.6%	26.2%	27.7%	28.5%	29.2%
Doubling time, days	3.4	3.3	3.2	3.0	2.8	2.8	2.7
Doubling time, hours	81	78	76	72	68	66	65
OMICRON variant	Generation time, days -->	3.5		Generation speed (G), Gen/ week		2.00
Reproduction number (R) >	2.80	2.90	3.00	3.20	3.40	3.50	3.60
Week-1	10.6	11.3	12.0	13.4	15.0	15.8	16.6
Week-2	83	95	108	138	173	193	215
Week-3	654	800	972	1,409	1,999	2,363	2,781
Week-4	5,127	6,727	8,748	14,431	23,110	28,953	36,048
Last week of Month-1	10,186	13,681	18,197	31,338	52,255	66,742	84,673
Last week of Month-2	76,447,762	139,176,285	248,336,459	748,225,094	2,109,963,722	3,464,633,004	5,610,893,312
Last week of Month-3	573,765,432,901	1,415,841,228,215	3,389,154,437,772	17,864,824,263,349	85,197,255,046,191	179,851,317,062,612	371,809,387,633,792
Week-to-week growth factor	7.8	8.4	9.0	10.2	11.6	12.3	13.0
Month-to-month growth factor	7,505	10,173	13,647	23,876	40,379	51,911	66,266
Day-to-day growth, %	34.2%	35.6%	36.9%	39.4%	41.9%	43.0%	44.2%
Doubling time, days	2.4	2.3	2.2	2.1	2.0	1.9	1.9
Doubling time, hours	57	55	53	50	48	46	45

Corona Table, page 4: Theoretical WEEKLY new infection rates originating from ONE infected person with OMICRON, DELTA, or the ORIGINAL VERSION of Corona.

CORONA TABLE							Page 5
THEORETICAL WEEKLY NEW COVID-19 INFECTIONS ORIGINATING FROM ONE INFECTED PERSON							
ORIGINAL version	Generation time, days -->		7.0	Generation speed (G), Gen/ week -->			1.00
Reproduction number (R) >	3.80	4.00	4.20	4.40	4.50	4.60	4.80
Week-1	3.8	4.0	4.2	4.4	4.5	4.6	4.8
Week-2	14	16	18	19	20	21	23
Week-3	55	64	74	85	91	97	111
Week-4	209	256	311	375	410	448	531
Last week of Month-1	325	406	502	614	677	745	895
Last week of Month-2	105,874	165,140	252,054	377,216	458,327	554,500	801,846
Last week of Month-3	34,449,804	67,108,864	126,543,772	231,677,999	310,286,356	412,906,588	718,019,247
Week-to-week growth factor	3.80	4.00	4.20	4.40	4.50	4.60	4.80
Month-to-month growth factor	325	406	502	614	677	745	895
Day-to-day growth, %	21.0%	21.9%	22.8%	23.6%	24.0%	24.4%	25.1%
Doubling time, days	3.6	3.5	3.4	3.3	3.2	3.2	3.1
Doubling time, hours	87	84	81	79	77	76	74
DELTA variant	Generation time, days -->		5.0	Generation speed (G), Gen/ week -->			1.40
Reproduction number (R) >	3.80	4.00	4.20	4.40	4.50	4.60	4.80
Week-1	7.4	8.0	8.5	9.0	9.3	9.5	10.1
Week-2	48	55	63	72	76	81	91
Week-3	313	386	471	570	626	685	816
Week-4	2,026	2,686	3,514	4,539	5,137	5,799	7,332
Last week of Month-1	3,778	5,130	6,865	9,063	10,365	11,820	15,244
Last week of Month-2	12,432,573	23,047,106	41,462,454	72,591,261	95,148,764	123,979,879	206,999,356
Last week of Month-3	40,918,041,714	103,541,316,015	250,438,270,760	581,429,744,634	873,425,229,886	1,300,415,250,790	2,810,816,538,031
Week-to-week growth factor	6.5	7.0	7.5	8.0	8.2	8.5	9.0
Month-to-month growth factor	3,291	4,493	6,040	8,010	9,180	10,489	13,579
Day-to-day growth, %	30.6%	32.0%	33.2%	34.5%	35.1%	35.7%	36.9%
Doubling time, days	2.6	2.5	2.4	2.3	2.3	2.3	2.2
Doubling time, hours	62	60	58	56	55	55	53
OMICRON variant	Generation time, days -->		3.5	Generation speed (G), Gen/ week -->			2.00
Reproduction number (R) >	3.80	4.00	4.20	4.40	4.50	4.60	4.80
Week-1	18.2	20.0	21.8	23.8	24.8	25.8	27.8
Week-2	263	320	385	460	501	545	641
Week-3	3,803	5,120	6,796	8,905	10,149	11,534	14,779
Week-4	54,919	81,920	119,880	172,410	205,518	244,058	340,500
Last week of Month-1	133,736	206,425	312,067	462,947	560,177	675,043	968,897
Last week of Month-2	14,159,241,271	34,089,178,019	78,657,792,414	174,630,786,145	256,744,065,848	374,311,018,171	776,905,514,385
Last week of Month-3	1,499,101,893,777,540	5,629,499,534,213,120	19,826,022,904,972,300	65,873,489,826,572,400	117,672,649,988,687,000	207,555,295,852,676,000	622,958,230,309,637,000
Week-to-week growth factor	14.4	16.0	17.6	19.4	20.3	21.2	23.0
Month-to-month growth factor	105,874	165,140	252,054	377,216	458,327	554,500	801,846
Day-to-day growth, %	46.4%	48.6%	50.7%	52.7%	53.7%	54.7%	56.5%
Doubling time, days	1.8	1.8	1.7	1.6	1.6	1.6	1.5
Doubling time, hours	44	42	41	39	39	38	37

Corona Table, page 5: Theoretical WEEKLY new infection rates originating from ONE infected person with OMICRON, DELTA, or the ORIGINAL VERSION of Corona.

CORONA TABLE					Page 6
THEORETICAL WEEKLY NEW COVID-19 INFECTIONS ORIGINATING FROM ONE INFECTED PERSON					
ORIGINAL version	Generation time, days -->	**7.0**	Generation speed (G), Gen/ week -->		**1.00**
Reproduction number (R) >	**5.00**	**5.50**	**6.00**	**6.50**	**7.00**	**7.50**
Week-1	5.0	5.5	6.0	6.5	7.0	7.5
Week-2	25	30	36	42	49	56
Week-3	125	166	216	275	343	422
Week-4	625	915	1,296	1,785	2,401	3,164
Last week of Month-1	1,069	1,615	2,355	3,331	4,593	6,193
Last week of Month-2	1,142,194	2,609,015	5,545,970	11,098,112	21,095,169	38,358,736
Last week of Month-3	1,220,703,125	4,214,198,260	13,060,694,016	36,972,058,910	96,889,010,407	237,572,640,181
Week-to-week growth factor	5.00	5.50	6.00	6.50	7.00	7.50
Month-to-month growth factor	1,069	1,615	2,355	3,331	4,593	6,193
Day-to-day growth, %	25.8%	27.6%	29.2%	30.7%	32.0%	33.4%
Doubling time, days	3.0	2.8	2.7	2.6	2.5	2.4
Doubling time, hours	72	68	65	62	60	58
DELTA variant	Generation time, days -->	**5.0**	Generation speed (G), Gen/ week -->		**1.40**
Reproduction number (R) >	**5.00**	**5.50**	**6.00**	**6.50**	**7.00**	**7.50**
Week-1	10.6	12.1	13.5	15.1	16.6	18.2
Week-2	101	131	166	207	253	306
Week-3	965	1,428	2,044	2,844	3,863	5,137
Week-4	9,182	15,534	25,116	39,089	58,889	86,263
Last week of Month-1	19,459	34,419	57,956	93,630	146,019	220,895
Last week of Month-2	338,485,014	1,067,414,903	3,047,048,700	7,999,987,485	19,558,643,160	44,966,755,978
Last week of Month-3	5,887,859,958,294	33,102,966,286,691	160,200,419,064,839	683,539,586,297,388	2,619,792,126,821,520	9,153,697,481,851,140
Week-to-week growth factor	9.5	10.9	12.3	13.7	15.2	16.8
Month-to-month growth factor	17,395	31,012	52,576	85,443	133,945	203,566
Day-to-day growth, %	38.0%	40.6%	43.1%	45.4%	47.6%	49.6%
Doubling time, days	2.2	2.0	1.9	1.9	1.8	1.7
Doubling time, hours	52	49	46	44	43	41
OMICRON variant	Generation time, days -->	**3.5**	Generation speed (G), Gen/ week -->		**2.00**
Reproduction number (R) >	**5.00**	**5.50**	**6.00**	**6.50**	**7.00**	**7.50**
Week-1	30.0	36	42	49	56	64
Week-2	750	1,081	1,512	2,060	2,744	3,586
Week-3	18,750	32,713	54,432	87,022	134,456	201,709
Week-4	468,750	989,583	1,959,552	3,676,671	6,588,344	11,346,130
Last week of Month-1	1,370,633	3,083,382	6,470,298	12,805,513	24,108,765	43,473,234
Last week of Month-2	1,565,529,736,337	8,044,590,684,216	35,884,078,352,367	142,117,018,759,215	508,578,473,451,993	1,667,578,272,010,720
Last week of Month-3	1,788,139,343,261,720,000	20,988,460,967,548,000,000	199,012,016,209,508,000,000	1,577,230,546,221,170,000,000	10,728,548,957,311,700,000,000	63,966,193,944,025,000,000,000
Week-to-week growth factor	25.0	30.3	36.0	42.3	49.0	56.3
Month-to-month growth factor	1,142,194	2,609,015	5,545,970	11,098,112	21,095,169	38,358,736
Day-to-day growth, %	58.4%	62.8%	66.9%	70.7%	74.4%	77.8%
Doubling time, days	1.5	1.4	1.4	1.3	1.2	1.2
Doubling time, hours	36	34	32	31	30	29

Corona Table, page 6: Theoretical WEEKLY new infection rates originating from ONE infected person with OMICRON, DELTA, or the ORIGINAL VERSION of Corona.

CORONA TABLE				Page 7
THEORETICAL WEEKLY NEW COVID-19 INFECTIONS ORIGINATING FROM ONE INFECTED PERSON				
ORIGINAL version	Generation time, days -->	7.0	Generation speed (G), Gen/ week -->	1.00
Reproduction number (R) >	8.00	8.50	9.00	9.50	10.00
Week-1	8.0	8.5	9.0	9.5	10.0
Week-2	64	72	81	90	100
Week-3	512	614	729	857	1,000
Week-4	4,096	5,220	6,561	8,145	10,000
Last week of Month-1	8,192	10,653	13,647	17,251	21,544
Last week of Month-2	67,108,864	113,491,679	186,252,345	297,580,575	464,158,883
Last week of Month-3	549,755,813,888	1,209,054,935,657	2,541,865,828,329	5,133,420,832,795	10,000,000,000,000
Week-to-week growth factor	8.00	8.50	9.00	9.50	10.00
Month-to-month growth factor	8,192	10,653	13,647	17,251	21,544
Day-to-day growth, %	34.6%	35.8%	36.9%	37.9%	38.9%
Doubling time, days	2.3	2.3	2.2	2.2	2.1
Doubling time, hours	56	54	53	52	51
DELTA variant	Generation time, days -->	5.0	Generation speed (G), Gen/ week -->	1.40
Reproduction number (R) >	8.00	8.50	9.00	9.50	10.00
Week-1	19.9	21.5	23.3	25.0	26.8
Week-2	365	431	504	585	673
Week-3	6,709	8,623	10,926	13,670	16,909
Week-4	123,310	172,518	236,808	319,574	424,731
Last week of Month-1	325,418	468,343	660,251	913,781	1,243,887
Last week of Month-2	97,991,167,211	203,722,564,681	406,237,896,447	780,486,256,522	1,450,266,042,471
Last week of Month-3	29,507,529,625,970,900	88,616,368,957,666,000	249,949,146,802,651,000	666,635,543,361,298,000	1,690,886,064,459,000,000
Week-to-week growth factor	18.4	20.0	21.7	23.4	25.1
Month-to-month growth factor	301,124	434,986	615,278	854,128	1,165,914
Day-to-day growth, %	51.6%	53.4%	55.2%	56.9%	58.5%
Doubling time, days	1.7	1.6	1.6	1.5	1.5
Doubling time, hours	40	39	38	37	36
OMICRON variant	Generation time, days -->	3.5	Generation speed (G), Gen/ week -->	2.00
Reproduction number (R) >	8.00	8.50	9.00	9.50	10.00
Week-1	72	81	90	100	110
Week-2	4,608	5,834	7,290	9,002	11,000
Week-3	294,912	421,520	590,490	812,470	1,100,000
Week-4	18,874,368	30,454,823	47,829,690	73,325,416	110,000,000
Last week of Month-1	75,497,472	126,843,642	206,947,050	328,904,846	510,574,772
Last week of Month-2	5,066,549,580,791,790	14,395,697,935,520,900	38,544,373,186,193,100	97,875,693,464,571,300	236,987,815,903,507,000
Last week of Month-3	340,010,386,766,614,000,000,000	1,633,791,935,959,750,000,000,000	7,178,979,876,918,530,000,000,000	29,125,905,177,792,600,000,000,000	110,000,000,000,000,000,000,000,000
Week-to-week growth factor	64	72	81	90	100
Month-to-month growth factor	67,108,864	113,491,679	186,252,345	297,580,575	464,158,883
Day-to-day growth, %	81.1%	84.3%	87.3%	90.3%	93.1%
Doubling time, days	1.2	1.1	1.1	1.1	1.1
Doubling time, hours	28	27	26	26	25

Corona Table, page 7: Theoretical WEEKLY new infection rates originating from ONE infected person with OMICRON, DELTA, or the ORIGINAL VERSION of Corona.